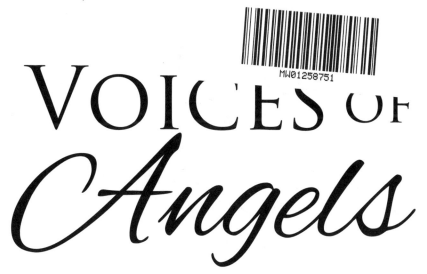

VOICES OF
Angels

DISASTER LESSONS
FROM KATRINA NURSES

VOICES OF
Angels
DISASTER LESSONS FROM KATRINA NURSES

BY GAIL TUMULTY
AND JOHN R. BATTY

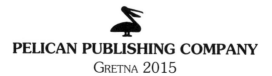

PELICAN PUBLISHING COMPANY
GRETNA 2015

*The word "Pelican" and the depiction of a pelican are
trademarks of Pelican Publishing Company, Inc., and are
registered in the U.S. Patent and Trademark Office.*

ISBN: 9781455621231
E-book ISBN 9781455621248

All photos by John Jones, John Penland and Tim Butcher, unless
otherwise noted.

Printed in the United States of America
Published by Pelican Publishing Company, Inc.
1000 Burmaster Street, Gretna, Louisiana 70053

This book is dedicated to Dr. Barbara Gail Tumulty

Dr. Barbara Gail Tumulty is one of the most important and influential persons in the history of nursing and the lives of thousands of people around the world. The patients she treated, the nurses she led, and the nurses she taught all owe her everlasting gratitude for changing their lives with her positive force.

She was the inspiration behind the creation of the Loyola Health Care System Management Program, in the Graduate School of Nursing. It was the first online program in the history of the university, and was founded with approximately $2 million in federal and state grants. Now in its eleventh year, the program has trained over 1,150 nurses from around the world to be managers. Loyola has benefited enormously in grants, prestige and international reputation because of Gail's work.

She was universally regarded as an outstanding nursing educator and mentor to her loyal students. Loyola recognized her importance to the Graduate School of Nursing and bestowed upon her the title of Emeritus when she retired in 2014. These magnificent accomplishments are the work of a quiet, brilliant young angel from Kansas.

As the coauthor of the book *Voices of Angels* I often marveled at her people skills, her persuasive smile and her native intelligence. It was one of the most fortunate and productive friendships in my life. Any success that may come from this project will not be the same without her here to enjoy it.

We wanted the true story of the nurses who are angels written and saved for history. We wanted young nurses to someday be inspired by the heroic actions taken by the nurse angels who worked in every Louisiana and Gulf Coast hospital and healthcare center in the wrath of Katrina.

And now, her friends, her colleagues and wonderful loving family feel she is with the angels, smiling down upon us.

— John R. Batty, RN, MSN, HCSM

Contents

Acknowledgments

My wife Jan has been an invaluable moral support in the process of this book. Without her encouragement and constructive criticism, this book would not have happened. I am deeply grateful to Mary Len Costa for her invaluable advice, assistance and encouragement. James Nolan's consistently high standards for the art and the craft of writing have been both an inspiration and a challenge for me and many other students. Carolyn Perry has been a wonderful resource for style, good writing, and the art of the craft.

Introduction

By John Batty, RN, MSN, HCSM

I am a nurse "raised up" in the Charity Hospital tradition. Killer hurricane named Katrina? Hah! We don't run. We stay to take care of the poor, we stay to be the last hope for everyone, and we stay because it is in our blood—or maybe you should be working somewhere else. We could not imagine leaving a patient to die; we stay to the bitter end, whatever that outcome might be. However, the two toughest women in my life looked me straight in the eye.

Miss Rita, 85, lived in the 1400 block of Polymnia St., in the Lower Garden District all her life. The first born of Sicilian immigrants, she had saved the down payment for her craftsman double from a clerk's salary. When the neighborhood went down and the grand old houses were converted to 18-unit tenement apartments, she became the rock of the neighborhood. And when it came back, the young professionals viewed her as the Sheriff of Polymnia Street.

Hurricane? Hah! She wouldn't think of leaving. When a hurricane threatened the year before, the feisty little lady came to us: "Can I borrow a life vest? I might have to swim for it."

My darling wife, Miss Kitten, had other ideas. She had been the curator of a French Quarter house museum built in 1832, and she knew the Mississippi River. Kitten was from Memphis and could recite the history of crevasses and floods when the levees split wide open in 1927, and flooded towns in Arkansas, Mississippi, and Louisiana. She knew the history.

"We're leaving," she said, "I'm not hanging around here when 22 feet of water is forecast for the front yard in 48 hours. I never saw anything like this in Memphis, and I'm not starting now. We're out of here tomorrow morning, do you hear me?"

As a veteran psych nurse, I filtered out the anxiety and focused on the positive. "But Kitten, the levees are modern, state-of-the-art engineering marvels designed by the US Army Corps of Engineers, and they haven't breached since the 1930s."

"Do you think Katrina and a 22-foot storm surge gives a damn?" she steamed, channeling her level best Scarlett O'Hara piercing voice.

"But Kitten, there is no mandatory evacuation. If it's up to me, I'd never leave New Orleans, besides, we're on high ground. Do you think Miss Rita is leaving? Certainly not! And besides, I can volunteer at Charity."

"Well, you can stay, but I'm leaving, and you and Miss Rita who love this sinkhole of a city so much can swim for it," she said.

On the earliest maps the city is called the Isle de Orleans. It is surrounded by subtropical swamps on the east and west, Lake Pontchartrain on the north and the Mississippi River to the south. It was an excellent home to insects of all kinds, snakes, alligators, disease, pestilence, natural disasters and calamity. When New Orleans became an international port, it just opened the door for more lethal problems.

In fact, the city has had a long list of perfect natural disasters such as yellow fever, malaria, flooding, fire, typhoid, cholera, venereal disease, hurricanes, and many imported disasters such as nutria, Formosan termites, red ants and killer bees. Yellow fever killed 41,000 residents in the 1800s, but that was merely the official number.[1]

The nutria hitchhiked from South America then burrowed into the levees and canal banks so much that the structures materially weakened. Jefferson Parish Sheriff Harry Lee sent his sharpshooters out at night to whack them, and the state put a $7 bounty on their pelts.[2]

Formosan termites arrived courtesy of the shipping industry, and promptly started eating creosote docks, French Quarter landmarks, Garden District mansions, and everything else.[3]

Levees have routinely failed throughout our history. Engineers have said levees are designed to fail at a certain level of stress that Mother Nature has always found. Before Katrina, residents of the Lakeview neighborhood near the 17th Street Canal had complained to the New Orleans Levee Board of leaks in the base of the levees causing puddles to form in yards. The board did nothing about it. "Oh, that was natural," the levee board told residents.[4] It was little surprise that the concrete and earthen 17th Street Canal failed spectacularly, sending a flood tide roaring into the city that reached rooftops across the city and into the Lower Ninth Ward.

If anyone knew this dicey history of disease, flood, and disaster, it was Miss Rita. When she knocked on the front door, we wondered what to expect. Would she give us her standard hurricane advice born of 85 years? Did she have a premonition to tell us?

"Jan, John, come out here on the porch and talk to me." The voice of the little Sicilian was strangely calm and reserved. The stainless steel in her character was showing.

"I'm going to tell you something I never thought I would say in my life—I'm leaving. Can I catch a ride to my relatives in Covington?" Her cool gaze told me all I needed to know. She had weighed the possibilities, she was leaving town for the first time in 85 years. I was hard aground between history and cold logic. It was time to make discretion the wiser part of valor.

"You're right, Miss Rita," Jan said, meeting her gaze, "we're leaving at noon and we are delighted to have you with us."

The car was packed, the engine was running and the air conditioner purring. I took one last set of pictures of the home we shared with Miss Rita. We had no idea what we would find when we returned, if indeed we managed to return to our home on Polymnia St.

Introduction

By Dr. Gail Tumulty, RN, BSN, MSN, CNAA

Like the million-plus residents of Southeast Louisiana, my husband Joe and I evacuated the city late on Saturday evening after the 10 p.m. news. We expected to return in a few days.

Mayor Ray Nagin shared the forecast from the National Hurricane Center that the levees in New Orleans were predicted to fail. Joe was not intimidated by this news, but I was ready to evacuate for the first time in our lives. Our children kept calling to encourage us to move to safer ground. We packed a few things "just in case." Due to the late hour, traffic was light and we drove easily north on I-55 toward Jackson, Mississippi. I insisted we keep going to our daughter's home in Columbia, Missouri. We arrived later that Sunday evening, staying there for two weeks when we heard that we were allowed to return to New Orleans.

We steered south and stopped for the night in Memphis. By the next day, the entrance into New Orleans was stopped by a second hurricane named Rita. We decided to reroute to Dallas where our youngest son, his wife and baby had rented an apartment. We stayed with them to share the baby's first birthday and then left again for New Orleans.

New Orleans was clearly decimated by the storm. Loyola University had been closed for the fall semester and students and faculty were not allowed at the school. The National Guard had taken over the campus with so many vehicles it looked like an Army base. Like most of the city, streets around Loyola narrowed to one lane, crowded by trees, building debris and garbage. Our home suffered roof damage, kitchen damage, with 3.5 feet of water in the lower level and other exterior damage.

The nursing graduate program, health care systems management, was fully online as well as on-campus. I was the coordinator and put our program back online as soon as the technology was available. Even students who could not attend class on-campus were welcomed to the online classes. No students were refused. Students appreciated the ability to keep up with their classes and finish their classes on time.

Loyola University New Orleans reopened in January 2006 when classes fully restarted. As students returned to class, it became clear they were in the later stages of shock. The students were seasoned nurses earning a master's degree in health care systems management. They worked in a variety of positions at area hospitals. Many were managers who shouldered a great deal of responsibility.

The stories they told were amazing to those who had not been in the hospitals. The nurses were kind enough to allow taping of their stories and shared what had happened in the five to six days that they spent in the hospitals caring for their patients and taking care of themselves.

This book will be a beginning of the things that these nurses shared. Some stories are about the horrors of the recovery of the hospitals. The lack of electricity, food and water threatened lives. It was and still is amazing to realize the realities that the nurses endured.

Into this moment of governmental chaos and incompetence, in stepped the perfect monster to thrash the City That Care Forgot.

Although many nurses said they would rather die than desert a patient to suffer alone, enough patients died at one hospital to spark investigations, grand juries, and an attorney general who wanted to find the truth. All he found was a quick exit for a Louisiana incumbent.

The Bible tells us much about angels on earth and in heaven. This book is about the angels who walk with us every day and lead us in caring for others. Those nurses who lost loved ones, who lost everything they owned, and everything in their futures, struggled on to care for their patients despite everything they suffered.

These women and men are the Nurse Angels of Katrina. And these are the legends of how they earned their wings.

Chapter 1

Katrina Is Born

Over 100,000 residents and visitors were stuck in the City That Care Forgot. It was the end of the August 2005, and the Social Security checks that many of these impoverished people depended upon for food and utilities had not been mailed. They were broke and going nowhere fast. The monster hurricane of a lifetime bore down on them with no mercy. The plans to bus folks out of town did not happen. The buses themselves were not moved to higher ground. Mayor Ray Nagin knew this. They flooded just like some of their riders.

Diehard New Orleanians seldom imagined leaving home for a hurricane. This time they did. The six-lane highway contraflow opened on Saturday, August 27, 2005 at 4 p.m. and worked so efficiently that it was closed Sunday at 6 p.m. In approximately 26 hours, over 1 million evacuees fled New Orleans and surrounding communities.[1]

The shake, rattle and roll of the city headed out of town. The birthplace of jazz hushed eerily. Natives accustomed to makin' groceries on Saturday were suddenly confronted with a surreal emptiness they never imagined. Even the French Quarter seemed to roll to a depressing stop. Stillness hung in the air like the hot humid blanket of August.

The evacuation of patients and seniors from public and private hospitals and senior centers was far more complicated. Evacuation wasn't even considered by most hospital leaders for the simple fact they were extremely limited in destinations. Where to flee? How to get there? How to pay for it?

New Orleans was the largest city with the largest concentration of doctors, specialists, and hospitals in the state. Even with one-way highway contraflow, the route to Baton Rouge was a seventy-five-mile parking lot, by ambulance or pick-up truck. Most evacuation helicopters could not reach Alexandria—much less Shreveport or Monroe, where hundreds of empty hospital beds awaited.

The time and money for moving thousands of patients would stun even the Pentagon. Simply ordering Charity Hospital staff to Code Grey hurricane watch cost an additional $600,000 per day in added staff expense.[2]

Transportation expenses could be astronomical for even a simple evacuation. An ambulance trip to the nearest hospital, Earl K. Long Hospital in Baton Rouge that could take Charity patients could easily exceed $1,000 per patient, for a 200-mile roundtrip, in 2005. There were simply not enough ambulances or staff in the state to move patients by ground.

Air evacuation was slow and expensive. In 2006 it started at

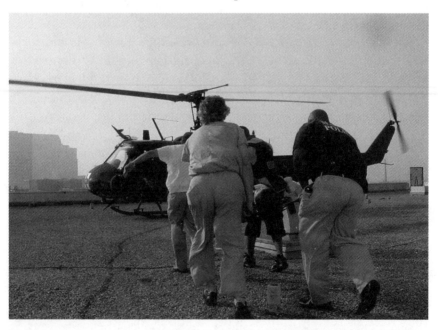

Helicopter evacuation mobilized Tuesday at University Medical Center. Other hospitals like Charity watched and waited in vain for promised help that did not come.

$12,000 per patient plus mileage. Acadian Ambulance Service helicopters could carry maybe two patients and an attendant on each trip. [3]

The rate for evacuating one patient could approach $15,000 depending on the length and destination of the trip. Public hospitals would be reimbursed by FEMA, but the private hospitals were not. Hospital administrators winced at the thought of a budget-busting evacuation.

Katrina defied decision-making. The speed and unpredictable path of hurricanes is legendary. The Department of Veterans Affairs Medical Center, for example, had a timetable that required evacuation decisions be made within 36 to 72 hours before storm landfall.[4]

It was a formula for disaster. Further complicating the decision was a state law that restricted the operations of ambulances in weather with winds less than 45 mph.

※※※※※

In New Orleans East, Pendleton Memorial Methodist Hospital was an attractive general hospital, served by a veteran staff of doctors and nurses. Its gleaming white exterior was a beacon for miles across the flat marshy eastern edge of the city, and it gave residents a sense of safety knowing it was near in time of need.

The Methodist Foundation that built the hospital sold its majority ownership in 2003 to Universal Health Services, based in King of Prussia, Pennsylvania. UHS installed the energetic Chief Executive Officer Larry Graham to lead its new acquisition.

Graham was closely monitoring the hurricane on Friday. Thinking Katrina was going ashore in Alabama or Florida, he decided to go fishing on the Saturday before Katrina mauled Louisiana, according to his trial testimony in 2010.[5]

Graham received no calls from the city or the state authorities. And when it became evident that the hurricane would hit the city, it was too late to evacuate, he later reported to the House Congressional Select Bipartisan Committee investigating the disaster.[6] He also testified that he called his corporate office for helicopters to evacuate the patients of Methodist Hospital on Tuesday after the storm came ashore. The helicopters did not arrive because, Graham reported, the helicopters and supplies were seized by FEMA.[7]

Nurses, doctors and emergency responders in states on the Gulf of Mexico and the Atlantic were well aware of hurricane season. They knew the bulk of patient care would fall directly on them. Most had all suffered personal losses in previous storm seasons. Betsy in 1965 and Camille in 1969 were deadly and dangerous hurricanes that lurked in the memories of coastal residents. Louisiana and Mississippi natives lived in fear due to the long histories of these tragic events.

The Medical Center of Louisiana was composed of two venerable old hospitals only a few blocks apart: Charity and University. Both were vital to the city.

Charity Hospital was founded in 1736 with a grant by a French shipbuilder Jean Louis. He died before he could see the hospital for the poor ever open.

Until Katrina, Charity served the poor for 250 years. The Sisters of Charity ran the hospital for a century. Many others stepped in—including Gov. Huey Long and the LSU Healthcare System to build Charity. First Gov. Kathleen Blanco then Gov. Bobby Jindal would make sure the Charity never reopened in the decade after Katrina. It was the second-oldest continuously operating hospital in the US. Bellevue Hospital in New York is only a month older. To predominantly poor, uninsured minorities, the hospital provided primary and specialized care to well over half the population.[8]

As a Level One Trauma Center, Big Charity was the go-to ER, and accounted for well over 80 percent of the uncompensated medical costs in the city.[9]

The street called Charity the *Big Free C*. Its ER was the destination of choice for crime victims, those suffering severe trauma such as spinal cord or brain injuries, and life-threatening accidents all over New Orleans and South Louisiana. If you got shot, stabbed or were ready to be born or die, you wanted Charity. Its trauma surgery suites were staffed by outstanding nurses, residents and surgeons. Over half of the poverty-level households in the city had family members suffering from chronic diseases such as asthma, hypertension, diabetes, chronic obstructive pulmonary disease, coronary artery disease and chronic kidney disease. Many were treated at Charity.[10]

The massive 18-story structure was completed in 1939 as a dream of the late Louisiana Gov. Huey Long. Assassinated in 1935, he did not live to see it completed for "every man a king." Its footprint covered almost all of a large double city block, and its art deco designs added a luster of glimmering beauty to Tulane Avenue in its heyday. Its three-foot thick walls of steel and reinforced concrete inspired the staff with a sense of confidence it would survive any hurricane. It was a commanding presence in the Depression era when it opened, and over the years the uninsured and poor population came to regard it as their savior in time of medical need.

The annual storm preparations and exercises at Charity and other South Louisiana hospitals gave the staff essential training that would help them survive in the days to come. Many hospitals divided staff into two groups. The Ready Team or A Team would ride out the storm in place. The Recovery Team or B Team had the task of returning after the storm. The two teams relied on a volunteer staffing system that seemed to work for local hospitals.

Ready Team Members Bring Families, Pets, Chicken

Many of the nurses who volunteered for the Ready Team had established a practice of gathering the members of their families who could not evacuate, bringing them into the hospital to stay until the storm passed.

At Charity, more members than the immediate family came. They brought with them appetites for New Orleans cuisine—and the gear to cook it on. Fried chicken, boudin sausage, fried catfish, red beans and rice.

At Ochsner Medical Center, just over the line in Jefferson Parish, some brought pets.

Families at Charity Hospital dragged barbecue pits, microwaves, iceboxes loaded with food, and generally moved into the hospital for the duration.

Families and evacuees at Pendleton complained they weren't receiving the same food as the staff, causing staff to advise them they could leave any time they pleased. But the snakes, alligators and nasty water surrounding the hospital gave the visitors second thoughts about striking out into the outside world.

Although this family-friendly practice made logistical planning difficult, it was much easier to find enough volunteer veteran staff to meet the hospital's needs when they were allowed to bring their families into the hospital. The practice of bringing families into the hospital to weather hurricanes was great for the nurses who brought the clan with them.

However, subsequent events changed the plan after 2005. The families proved to be so much of a diversion to the hospital staff and its resources that the Joint Commission of the Accreditation of Hospitals recommended the policy end after 2005.

John Jones, the director of nursing at Charity, had grown up in Florida, and regarded storms as a routine display of nature. "I kinda liked the lightning, the wind and all of the rain, as long as nobody got hurt, and when it was over, the sun came out again."[11]

But much of the coast of Florida was above sea level. When hurricane storm surges rolled inland, floodwaters returned to the Gulf, Atlantic, bays, bayous and rivers.

New Orleans was built on swamps, bayous, old sandbars, and sediment deposited by the Mississippi River over millions of years. Half of the land in the city was anywhere from 2 to 15 feet below sea level. The Crescent City was surrounded by water. It was Lake Pontchartrain on the north, the Mississippi River on the south and vast swamps on the east and west. When the famously poor levees were built to keep hurricane storm surge out, some simply raised the edges of the bowl, and retained the floodwater. Even though the city had massive pumps and efficient drainage canals, a thunderstorm often resulted in street flooding and feverish pumping

"Preparing for hurricanes had become so routine to most of us," said Jones. "You collected all of the things you would need for a short trip, loaded up the family and moved into Charity. The supplies of water, food, and medical disposables were moved from the warehouse into the hospital and placed where they were most likely to be used throughout the hospital. We had done it before and everyone knew what their responsibilities entailed and where their families were staying," Jones said. "We knew the routine, and we were all proud Charity nurses."[12]

John Jones was a veteran US Navy nurse who had served in the Pacific during Vietnam caring for wounded soldiers and airmen being transported back to the States. He was of average stature, but in his eyes one saw courage, determination, and the ability to fearlessly lead his nurses in the worst of times. He did not frighten easily. In the private sector, he had paid his dues in climbing the ladder to nurse executive. His calm demeanor and the air of confidence earned from wartime experience made him the perfect leader between senior hospital administrators and line staff. He fit the role of the nurse CEO.

The annual hurricane preparations at Charity had been in place for as long as any nurse could remember. The yearly exercises had engendered an assured attitude of survival. Many nurses proudly told people if you were "raised up" at Charity, you had confidence that you could survive anything. Monster Hurricane Katrina? So what?

But this hurricane was different. Could it be the tragic killer disaster everyone feared? They called it *The Big One*. The old veteran nurses kept respect. The city had a history of evading killers like Camille. Somehow, this hurricane was different. Maybe their time had come. As the hurricane drew a bead on the city, many braced for the dreaded "worst case scenario,"as it was famously known to the National Weather Service.

While over a million people already fled South Louisiana, many nurses and doctors realized the peril for those left behind. "It was kind of strange to be the only one on the interstate coming into town," said a Ready Team member enroute to the hospital, "when it looked like everyone else on the other side of the interstate seemed to be headed out of town."[13]

These moments made some nurses feel the eye of the killer was headed directly for them.

It is the duty of nurses to remain calm in life-threatening events, otherwise your patient could be lost. But some were scared stiff and not afraid to admit it. The ER nurses who had seen every kind of injury and trauma the devil could imagine had not seen a direct hit on the city since Hurricane Betsy in 1965. The city was overdue and they knew it.

Lucy, a veteran of the ER, was nervous about the storm, "I don't know what it was—I mean I've been on the Ready Team for years—but I never had this feeling about a storm before." Lucy asked that her name be changed for this interview. She spoke softly, earnestly. "I just knew this was *The Big One*. It was headed right for us. I was worried about my daughter more than anything else, so I found her a hotel on Canal Street and told her to just sit tight."[14]

Lucy is a devout, caring person who has lived in the sometimes horrific atmosphere of a big city ER, seeing the worst that man and machines can do to another human being. The ugly possibilities swirled in her mind as she thought about the Sunday night meeting they all faced with the hurricane called Katrina.

✕✕✕✕✕

It was after midnight on Sunday and the traffic was still inching on I-10 out of town. Katrina seemed to be headed directly for New Orleans, fulfilling the worst nightmares of many residents in the Big Easy and the Gulf Coast. Over 100,000 residents stayed behind to endure the killer storm. Katrina had grown to an enormously powerful Category 5 storm, and the TV weather reports had the monster aimed directly for New Orleans.

CNN correspondent John Zarrella, reporting from the French Quarter in New Orleans on Sunday night, August 28, 2005, said, "It's that calm before the storm, that eerie feeling...a light, light breeze, the wind barely moving. A little bit of a drizzle."[15]

Early Monday morning, the outlying feeder bands of the hurricane lashed South Louisiana with rain, and the NWS reported 55-foot high waves and winds over 175 mph in the eye of the storm. The massive hurricane covered an area 1,000 miles by 1,400 miles and pushed a 28-foot storm surge ahead of it, crushing everything in its path.[16]

At 6:30 a.m. the storm surge poured over the levees protecting New Orleans East from Lake Pontchartrain and within a few hours flooded the entire region, including Pendleton Memorial Methodist Hospital. Surprised nurses in the ER watched as a trickle of rain water suddenly grew to a torrent, announcing the huge levees only

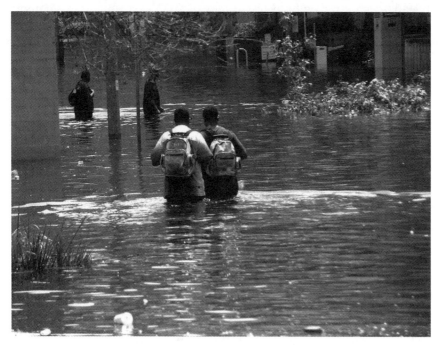

Residents who could not get out in time and those who need medical care converge at New Orleans hospitals. Some walk in, some wade in.

a few hundred yards away had been overtopped by raging storm surge. The destructive killer winds on the left side of the eye swept across the overloaded Lake Pontchartrain driving million of tons of water at the levees, then over the top. New Orleans East was doomed in minutes.

Pendleton had endured a miserable night of high winds, storm damage, broken windows, nurses scrambling to protect patients, staff and families. In the early morning light director of nursing Carol Beck-McCullogh realized the terrible impact of the rapidly rising water. She quickly turned to the staff and ordered them to move the ER to the next floor up. Patients, families, equipment— everything had to move before the rising water caught them. In seconds Pendleton would be surrounded by floodwaters soon teeming with snakes, alligators, and refugees trying to survive.

Suddenly, it seemed the hand of God intervened. The hurricane began to slightly wobble on its course, suggesting the city might avoid a direct hit. The massive eye of the storm was 30 miles wide, and it now directed its fury on a path slightly to the east of New Orleans, throwing its most intense and dangerous side directly toward the coast of Mississippi and Alabama, but sparing the city a paralyzing direct hit.

Katrina weakened to a Category 4 as it closed on the Louisiana coast and it came ashore at Buras, Louisiana, 65 miles south southeast of New Orleans, at 6:10 a.m. It destroyed everything in its path with sustained winds of 140 mph, gusts up to 200 mph, and a 21- foot storm surge. The killer ravaged a twenty-mile wide section of the Mississippi River levee below Port Sulphur, then jumped the mighty river on a course due north. The powerful right side of the hurricane smashed the Mississippi Gulf Coast for hours.

"The Water's Up to My Neck and I Can't Swim!"

"When the water hit the Lower Ninth Ward, it went from nothing to as high as 14 feet within 23 minutes," testified New Orleans Police Department Superintendent Warren J. Riley. [17]

When he walked into the Communications Section to get a report, he found almost every dispatcher and 911 operator crying.

"Chief, you have to listen in on the calls," a dispatcher said. He heard panicking mothers, fathers and children begging for help:
"I can't swim."
"My babies can't swim."
"My husband has drowned—please help me!"
"The water's up to my neck and I can't swim!"
"Oh my God, the wind just blew my husband off the roof!"
"God please help me!"[18]

The New Orleans Police Department fielded over six hundred 911 phone calls in 23 minutes but officers were powerless to help in winds over 100 mph.[19]

In the next few hours, the NOPD would see most of its stations flooded or destroyed, most of its equipment ruined and useless.

The New Orleans Fire Department suffered a similar fate of near total destruction, flooding and lost equipment.

The Louisiana National Guard headquarters was destroyed by a tsunami that flooded its trucks and equipment then swept a flood of water into its historic compound.

The modern FBI headquarters on the Lakefront was flooded and destroyed. The Coast Guard station on the Lakefront was washed away.

But the two most important organizations of men, women and machines had the foresight and experience to protect their assets and prepare for the most important mission of their lives. The Louisiana Department of Wildlife and Fisheries and the Coast Guard were experts in rescue at sea. The wildlife agency protected its patrol boats before the storm hit then prepared to launch shallow water *bateau* boats into the rapidly flooding city. In the most strategic action of the disaster, the Coast Guard moved helicopters to bases west and east of the storm for protection. The birds were poised to operate as soon as the hurricane blew inland.

Bordering the west side of New Orleans, the 17th Street Canal is the largest drainage outlet with the greatest pumping power in the city. A levee failure on this canal would be catastrophic because the massive pumps would have no place to send the floodwaters.

The concrete retaining walls of the canal toppled over. The torrent of water rushed from Lake Pontchartrain on the north side of the city into the fashionable neighborhoods of Lakeview, then further south to Mid-City.[20]

The Lakeview neighborhood was a lovely section of modern brick veneer houses built in the 1950s and later. The lovely postwar construction was favored in a community of older houses, but it had one tragic characteristic—the 17th Street Canal bordered on the west. As the retaining wall collapsed like dominoes, larger and larger waves from Lake Pontchartrain pushed into the city. The waves of water tossed aside wooden houses and simply swept the modern brick houses off their foundations. Entire blocks washed away in seconds. Lake Pontchartrain would pour in for the next four days, eventually covering everything with 4 to 12 feet of water.

At 7:45 a.m., two massive sections of the floodwall collapsed on the east side of the Industrial Canal, sending a torrential tidal wave into the lower Ninth Ward, Arabi, and Chalmette. The storm surge swept a 300-foot barge into the Lower Ninth Ward and flooded a large section of the city.[21]

Houses swept along with the torrent, only to be found blocks away, completely destroyed. Barely 45 minutes later the surge rolled over the secondary levee protecting St. Bernard Parish, and put its only hospital, Chalmette General Hospital, out of operation. Patients, families and staff quickly scurried to the second floor as the water rushed into the hospital.

Lindy Boggs Hospital was the next victim. The destruction and overtopping of levees and floodwalls in New Orleans continued with a vicious force. At 9:45 a.m., the 17th Street Canal floodwaters reached Mid-City, inundating Lindy Boggs Hospital. Although the flooding had begun early that morning, it was not reported in the media until much later in the day. [22]

Hurricane Katrina had devastated New Orleans. Few people would understand the depth and severity of the damage until later Monday. Even though the hurricane marched rapidly north, the tidal surge from Lake Pontchartrain continued to pour into the city for four more days until it reached the level of the lake on the north and the Gulf of Mexico on the south.[23]

In all of the other disastrous hurricanes in US history, the water drained away, but this hurricane was different. This time, the water stayed. Satellite weather images showed a city that was 80 percent underwater with all of its important pumping stations deeply submerged and fatally wounded.

John Jones and most of the nurses at Charity exhaled relief that the monster had moved north. The balmy skies that followed bore no hint of the trauma to come to the city and everyone who did not evacuate. The Ready Team thought Charity had dodged another hurricane, and they would be going home in a day or two.

When the floodwater climbed the ER ramp, people realized this hurricane was not going away quietly.

They had no idea of the coming ordeal at the *Big Free C*. And every other New Orleans hospital, retirement home and clinic.

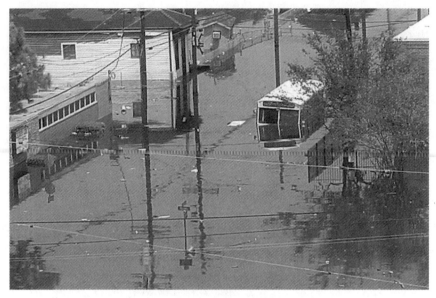

Over 80 percent of New Orleans flooded by Tuesday after Katrina hit. Water poured into the city for the next four days.

Chapter 2

Axes in the Attic

Forty years before Hurricane Katrina, the rising flood waters of Hurricane Betsy caught hundreds of Ninth Ward residents unprepared, forcing them to flee up to their attics. Many attics had no access to the roof and dozens of unprepared people died. In the grisly aftermath of Betsy, rescuers found the pitiful bodies of the people trapped in their attics with no way to get out. The terrible event started an urban legend: *Keep an axe in the attic if you want to survive a bad storm.*

The bad dreams of lost loved ones made it easy for native New Orleanians to be prepared. But in 2005 later hospital administrators did not know about the events of Betsy and could not imagine the levees would fail. They were supplied with food, water, generators, and the illusion that they were safe. The hospitals were made of concrete and steel able to withstand 150 mph winds, weren't they? If the water rose, they could go to the second floor, couldn't they? Nobody could imagine the catastrophic failure of the levees would allow floodwaters to rush into the city four days after the storm had passed. And then survive for an extended period of time without running water, electricity and air conditioning? The specter of misery was totally beyond imagination unless you had lived in the Ninth Ward.

✖✖✖✖✖

US Coast Guard Capt. Bruce Jones had evacuated his three HH-65 rescue aircraft 150 miles west of New Orleans. Monday morning as the hurricane roared ashore, Capt. Jones was plotting a rescue mission, but the conditions looked terrible. The tail end of the storm had limited visibility, strong winds, and possibly torrential rain. Accustomed to foul weather, Capt. Jones led his three rescue craft southeast from Houma that afternoon.[1]

Bobbie Moreau, her daughter Tasha, and Tasha's four month old preemie, lived in the town of Nairn, near Buras,, where the hurricane came ashore. They were forced to stay at home because she could not evacuate. She told the US Senate Committee investigating Katrina that swiftly rising water chased her upstairs in her home, "I shut the door upstairs, I guess, thinking I could shut the water out," she recalled. [2]

"From then on it was a nightmare. I held the baby at the foot of the bed fanning her. The pressure was awful: we thought the windows were going to pop. We got on our knees and prayed and begged God to save us. Then I felt the water under me on the second floor. I got up and walked to the window and the water was right under the window. My legs felt like Jell-O, I staggered. My daughter screamed, 'Mama, what's wrong?' I knew at that moment we were going to die."[3]

A mother's survival instinct emerged. Bobbie ripped the canopy from the bed, tied knots for her and Tasha to grip, and used a belt to make a life jacket for the baby. The water was surging through the house, now halfway up the bed, and the three were forced to climb out into the hurricane force wind onto the roof of the house with their three dogs. The winds unexpectedly calmed, "The eye of the hurricane was on us," said Bobbie. She knew this was their chance to find a way to survive, and told her daughter, "You will have to swim and get a boat, I am too weak."[4] The water had snakes, dead animals, and oil floating by them, Tasha said, "Mama, I'm scared." Bobbie told her, "We'll die if you don't."[5]

Bobbie watched her daughter swim out of sight. The wind grew, signaling the back of the eyewall with its ripping fierce winds. Fearing a new onslaught of hurricane force wind, she called her daughter, but heard no answer. She cried and prayed, and for a moment, she feared her daughter had drowned. She heard a boat's motor fire up, and soon saw her daughter coming to rescue her mother and baby.[6]

They huddled in the bottom of the boat, calling out Mayday on Channel 16, and they all prayed for rescue.[7]

Their prayers were answered once again. At 2:50 p.m. that afternoon, the Coast Guard responded to Bobbie's Mayday from the small boat in the middle Port Sulphur.[8]

Commander David Johnston, part of Capt. Jones's flight, heard the call and homed on its signal. While Cmdr. Johnson fought to stabilize his aircraft in 60-knot winds, rescue swimmer Laurence "Noodles" Nettles, was lowered 100 feet to save the lives of Bobbie Moreau and her brave little family.[9]

They became the first persons rescued by the Coast Guard, who would eventually rescue 33,554 people from the flooding of Katrina.[10]

Although her family was alive for the moment, their problems were far from over.

⨯⨯⨯⨯⨯

Approximately 6:30 a.m. the storm surge roared into New Orleans East, stranding Pendleton Memorial Methodist Hospital and flooding most of the area with two to twelve feet of water.

New Orleans Police Officer Chris Abbott was suddenly confronted with water rapidly rising in his house. He grabbed his police radio and his service weapon and ran up the steps to the attic. The water seemed to follow quickly, and Abbott radioed for help. The water quickly reached his chest. "I'm getting tired. I don't know if I'm going to make it."[11]

Captain Jimmy Scott radioed back to Abbott, telling him he could survive, and to find the attic vent and hang on. The radio went silent. Abbott had been wounded twice in the line of duty, and was well-known and liked in the police department. Fellow officers feared he would become another drowning-in-the-attic story, but the plucky Abbott radioed back. "I'm near the attic vent." Capt. Scott told him to punch it out. Abbott's reply stunned officers, "I don't think I'm going to make it. I'm getting very tired."[12]

He then started thanking everyone on the department for all
that they had done for him.

Capt. Scott asked Abbott if he had his police weapon and all
of his rounds. Abbott said he had his gun and 45 rounds. Capt.
Scott instructed him to carefully fire each round around the base
of the attic vent, "Shoot them all." The radio went silent for about
five minutes. Officers listened. Finally Abbott replied, "I'm halfway
out. I'm going to make it."[13]

✻✻✻✻✻

After decades of watching water drain after hurricanes passed,
New Orleans residents were stunned to see it suddenly rise. And it
was just the beginning of four days of rising water.

By the end of the day only two hospitals were still operating in New
Orleans. Children's Hospital was on high ground near the Mississippi
levee, and the venerable Touro Infirmary, one of the oldest hospitals
in the city, was on the high side of St. Charles Avenue.

"We were ordered to close the Friday after Katrina hit," said Paula
Fortier, Touro's archivist, "but we could have stayed open." The
hospital was safe enough that the New Orleans Police Department
had set up a substation in the hospital, and Touro was in sound
condition. "The order to close could have come from the mayor's
office," she added.

Elsewhere on the East Bank of the Mississippi River in Jefferson
Parish, Ochsner Medical Center and East Jefferson General Hospital
were two sprawling full-service hospitals that were prepared for the
storm. Ochsner had the distinct advantage of being on the natural
levee of the river, the highest ground in the suburban parish.
Floodwaters neared Ochsner but it did not flood. The center had
enough emergency generators to power emergency fans for nearly
all patients, an artesian well when the municipal water and power
failed and was well-stocked. East Jefferson Hospital was a 450-bed
center that suffered damaged and continued operating.

The 450-bed West Jefferson Medical Center was largest hospital on the West Bank of Jefferson Parish, and continued to stay open.

John Jones noted with satisfaction that the water had receded as the storm blew north, and the streets seemed to dry in the August heat. A few hours into the afternoon, he noticed that the water had returned. "It was dry at one moment, then a few inches appeared, then it rose quickly and seemed to keep on rising the rest of the day," said Jones. "At first, we didn't know that the levees had broken, and then the news started coming in and we all began to realize that we were looking at an entirely new situation."[14]

Medical Center of Louisiana at a Glance

—Founded in 1736 as a hospital for the poor, the medical center was comprised of the venerable old Charity Hospital and the newer University Hospital. Its ER is renowned for its excellent care of emergencies and trauma victims.

—New Orleans natives called it the *Big Free C* or simply "Charity." Charity was only a month younger than the oldest hospital in the US, Bellevue Hospital in New York City.

—The main building was completed in 1939 and had the capacity for 2,680. At that time it was the second largest hospital in the country.

—Charity has always been known to serve the poor and the most critical, as the Level 1 Trauma Center in South Louisiana. Gov. Huey Long focused on Charity in his "every man a king" oratory to help the poor, yet he was assassinated in 1935 before he could see it completed.

—The impressive cast aluminum artwork over the main entrance was designed by artist Enrique Alferez. It is called *Louisiana at Work and Play*.

※※※※※

Jean Baptiste Le Moyne, Sieur de Bienville, who founded the city of New Orleans in 1718, would not be surprised to see that over 80 percent of the city had flooded in 2005. On the early maps of the city the surrounding environment consisted of bayous, swamps, and thick jungle mostly below sea level.

The fashionable upper middle class neighborhood of Lakeview

is a good example. On maps showing the depth of the flooding due to the collapse of the 17th Street Canal, parts of Lakeview are as much as 15 feet under water. The great disparity in depth indicates old bayous, marsh and islands located there before Lakeview was pumped out and developed in the 1930s. It was a simple demonstration of local geography when media pundits noticed the striking similarity of a map showing the Hurricane Katrina flooding to a map of 1825.

The bottom line of vast flooding is that the New Orleans, state and federal leaders knew about it, planned for it, but failed to adequately prepare for it despite clear and present indications of danger.

Hurricane Betsy in 1965 delivered indisputable proof of the consequences of a levee failure. The Industrial Canal levee broke on the east, and then flooded the impoverished Lower Ninth Ward with five to nine feet of water. Four years later Camille stormed ashore in Pass Christian—about 30 miles east of New Orleans—as a Category 4 storm, one of the most powerful in history. Although a very compact hurricane, it had an estimated storm surge of 22 to 24 feet, and caused 262 deaths on the Mississippi Coast.

The worst-case storm for the city had been recognized and contemplated for so long that it earned the name the "New Orleans Scenario." The event was predicted to be a Cat 3 or stronger storm that would slug the city with a storm surge that would destroy or overtop the protective levees. The resulting flood would fill the saucer-shaped Crescent City with up to 15 feet of water that might take up to six months to drain and dry out.

The Hurricane Pam preparedness exercise in 2004 was to build a plan to respond to the devastation of a Category 3 hurricane hitting New Orleans. The long-range goal was a detailed paper describing the actions of local, state and federal agencies, which would be titled the "New Orleans Metropolitan Area Catastrophic Hurricane Plan.[15]

A priority of the analysis was to approximate the number and location of potential evacuees and to analyze current evacuation plans of the different agencies involved in the exercise. The event included over 300 participants from 15 federal agencies, state agencies, 13 parish agencies, five volunteer agencies, FEMA Region VI, and FEMA Headquarters.

Although the exercise covered many issues revolving around such a disaster, it failed to address massive nursing home and hospital evacuations required by rising water.

On August 27, 2005, barely two days before the landfall of Katrina, the exercise contractor finally delivered the Hurricane Pam draft plan to the city and FEMA[16]

It immediately became a hot topic at FEMA. The draft was widely circulated in the hours before Katrina hit South Louisiana.

Its predictions became painfully true:

Multiple levees were overtopped, flooding over 80 percent of the city, thousands of people were displaced for months, hospitals were overcrowded, generators failed throughout the city, and many first responders were incapacitated. But it did not predict a fatal failure in the levee system.

Low-lying New Orleans East and Chalmette in St. Bernard Parish were the first parts of the region where flooding was confirmed. Three canals located on the northern side of the city proved to be another fatal path.

Fire Captains Paul Hellmers and Joe Fincher, of Fire Engine 18, were stationed at Lake Marina Towers, an 18-story condominium on the Lakefront. The water seemed to be rising quickly, and it was coming from the direction of the 17th St. Canal.[17]

At 8:26 a.m., Helmers radioed the Fire Department Emergency Operations Center (EOC), "Water has risen eighteen inches over the past half hour in Lakeview. A levee may have broken or water may be pouring over the levee."[18]

The probability of the source of the water pointed to the nearby 17th Street Canal. The Marina Towers had a sweeping panoramic view of the entire lakefront and an excellent view of the three major canals that drained rainwater from the city into Lake Pontchartrain. Hellmers and Fincher led a small squad to the roof then reported to the EOC that the levee had breached. As they videotaped the damaged levee, Hellmers is heard saying, "You can see that the wall is gone, you can see the water pouring through, it looks like about a two-hundred-foot section of wall that's gone! The water is continuing to rise very slowly." He later told the *New Orleans Times Picayune*, "We knew it was all over, the entire city was going to flood."[19] The surging water roaring in from Lake Pontchartrain would continue to widen the breach and pour into the city for four days, sweeping away the houses in front of it, and destroying most of the property in that section of Lakeview.

✕✕✕✕✕

Hospitals built in the last hundred years are not designed to withstand flooding, high winds and power failure. Hospitals have huge demands for electricity, plumbing, refrigeration, oxygen lines, specialized evacuation lines, air treatment systems and sprinkler systems. All expensive and complicated to construct. An efficient design can be a weakness for disaster. [20]

Memorial Herman Hospital in Houston was a state-of-the-art hospital that was knocked out of service in 2004 by a thunderstorm. The floodwater water quickly drained away, and the generators were high and dry, Yet, the rainwater had poured down a truck loading ramp like it was a funnel—then rising high enough to destroy the electrical switching equipment.[21]

Poor planning for emergency generators would cause misery and death in Katrina.

Louisiana State Medical Director Dr. Jimmy Guidry later explained to the US Senate committee investigating Katrina that the state simply required that generators are present and functioning—not that they are installed at any particular level.

The same with critical switches. The location of the electrical switching equipment that would transfer the power from the generators throughout a hospital was not required to be installed at any particular distance above the ground or sea level.

Both vague standards resulted in a recipe for failure when rising floodwater shorted out the electrical switching systems that route power throughout the hospital. The absence of one sound standard for installing generators and electrical systems above the flood zone resulted in the destruction of the backup power systems in every South Louisiana hospital that suffered power failure.

⁕⁕⁕⁕⁕

Charity Hospital was one of the first institutional victims of flooded electrical switching equipment. The switching circuits located in the basement were destroyed as rising water flushed in.

Baptist Memorial Hospital was located in one of the lowest parts of Uptown New Orleans. It succumbed to flood waters that knocked out the electrical systems and the generators at once on the bottom floor and basement. Baptist began as Southern Baptist Hospital in 1926 and later separated from the Southern Baptist Convention.

Lindy Boggs Hospital in Mid-City suffered the same fate. This hospital conducted critical organ transplants and was fully occupied before evacuation. Tenet Healthcare operated Lindy Boggs Hospital, honoring the ambassador and member of Congress, after buying Mercy-Baptist Medical Center and changing names.

The healthcare workers, patients and families were marooned with typical South Louisiana August hot house levels of near 100 degrees and almost 100 percent humidity. Some windows opened, most did not. Later, Charity staff punched windows open. The same at other hospitals.

Even if the hospitals had working generators, they were designed for emergency power to run vital medical equipment. Generators were not powerful enough to run the air conditioning and refrigeration systems. But to their coming agony, the patients and healthcare workers would not be rescued quickly. Coast Guard protocol called for those in the most immediate danger—refugees clinging to roofs and flotsam—to be the first rescued.[22]

Katrina roared north, across New Orleans, Lake Pontchartrain and the Northshore of mostly suburban St. Tammany, Tangipahoa and mostly rural Washington Parish.

In New Orleans, 100,000 people were marooned on roofs, trapped in attics, clinging to anything that floated, and swimming in a sea of water that the media called a "toxic soup."[23]

Oil, sewage, toxic waste and chemicals from cars, truck, industrial storage and tens of thousands of homes quickly mixed with the rising saline lake water. And the bodies. Humans, animals, fish. To these stranded souls looking death in the face, rescue and evacuation was their only hope.

The rock-solid construction of the *Big Free C* was a comfort to both patients and staff—until the power died and the air conditioning failed. Everything about the building that added to its strength now conspired to turn it into hell. The heavy steel construction, concrete walls, and windows that had been painted shut for decades now trapped dead air and stench inside. The sealed environment grew hotter by the second.

Despite the misery of the conditions in a hospital, the huge buildings appeared to be an oasis of hope and safety in a sea of poison and danger. Refugees wading through the toxic soup were waved

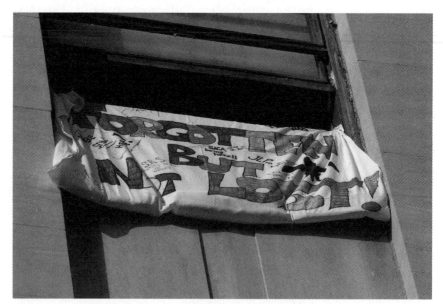

Charity Hospital bed sheets carry pleas and proclaim staff pride.

away from the already crowded hospitals. Those who were fortunate enough find something to float their way to higher ground received the same treatment. Nobody knew when the water would stop rising.

The saviors of thousands of helpless survivors came in aluminum jonboats and fiberglass fishing boats commandeered by volunteers, firemen, and emergency responders. Known as the Sportsman's Paradise, Louisiana's rich fishing waters have made bateaus, pirogues, and skiffs, as common as cattle in Texas. Fishermen and boaters launched their rigs and started pulling people out of the water, off rooftops, and moving them to the nearest high ground.

The same intrepid firemen, led by Captains Paul Hellmers and Joe Fincher, who first reported the break in the 17th Street Canal, early Monday morning, started looking for boats that looked like they would float. While the wind and rain was continuing to pound Lakeview that morning, they cranked up three fishing boats, and rescued people from rooftops, plucking them out of the water and moving them to higher ground.[24]

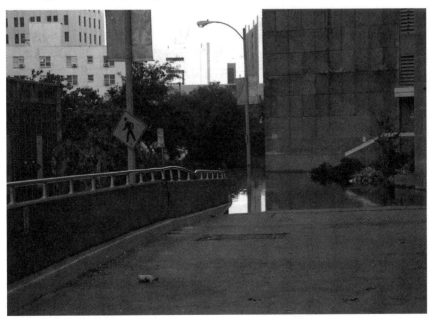

Floodwaters race up the ramp.

Meanwhile the 17th Street Canal breach widened, allowing a far larger torrent water to continue to pour into the city. The tsunami from the canal swept houses from foundations, then pulverized and destroyed everything in its path as it roared toward Mid-City.

The Louisiana Department of Wildlife and Fisheries was an important part of the Hurricane Pam exercise. They staged 60 of their small patrol boats before Katrina made landfall. They were ready, willing, and determined to launch into the flooded city as soon as conditions permitted on the day of landfall.

Wildlife agents launched boats by 4 p.m. and jump-started their rescue efforts. They had staged their boats in strategic locations on high ground that allowed them to launch as soon as possible, much to the great relief of the thousands of people they would pull from the flood.

"We put two officers in a boat, one guy to operate the boat and another guy with a flashlight to give him direction," said Lt. Col. Keith LaCaze, LDWF. "Most of our communication at this point was by voice. And they would go out and like I said, it wasn't any problem to find people. There were people everywhere, people were everywhere, every house, people on the porches, people shouting from windows and you would just go to it and load up the people that you could and take them and tell them, We'll be back for the rest of you...."[25]

The Coast Guard 8th district headquarters, located on the New Orleans Lakefront conducted search-and-rescue throughout the Gulf of Mexico and major inland waterways starting with the Mississippi River and Lake Pontchartrain. The Coast Guard prepared for Katrina by evacuating dependents, air crews, support personnel, and the vital helicopters. They relocated their rescue headquarters 200 miles north to Alexandria, Louisiana.[26]

Their critical rescue helicopters were strategically located west, north and east of the expected landfall in order to be able to respond rapidly. Their liaisons with the state and federal government were well connected for communications and quick response.

The Louisiana National Guard headquarters in Jackson Barracks was located just north of Chalmette in Arabi. It is a 100-acre base featuring 14 historic garrison structures built in the 1840s. When Katrina struck, the National Guard was stretched thin because its combat brigade remained deployed in Iraq. Elements of the Guard were deployed in the Superdome and several hospitals throughout New Orleans to maintain security. Over 20,000 people flooded into the Superdome, which flooded itself. The roof failed. Six died at the Superdome of various causes and rumors incorrectly spiked higher.

The storm surge rolled over the back levee on the gulf side of Arabi and made a beeline for the headquarters. A raging wave of floodwaters quickly overran the trucks and rescue vehicles of the Guard, and sent officers and men scampering to the second floor of the buildings.[27]

The Louisiana National Guard had much of its equipment and supplies destroyed by the floodwaters. Lt. Gen. H. Steven Blum, Chief, National Guard Bureau, reacted swiftly to send in materials and vital reinforcements. Within 24 hours of landfall 9700 National Guard soldiers and airmen were in New Orleans, and within 96 hours the National Guard deployed over 30,000 troops to assist in the rescue and security activities.

Gen. Blum and Gen. Clyde A. Vaughn called Louisiana State Adjutant Gen. Benny Landreneau. as the storm passed the city, asking him what help they could send. But Gen. Landreneau was stranded in the Superdome surrounded by water too deep for trucks. His armory in Chalmette was flooded.[28]

The National Guard and other military branches mobilized fast and stayed long. The US Army, Navy, Air Force, Marines and almost every state agency in the country that could send help to Louisiana did so with urgency.

⁑⁑⁑⁑⁑

John, an experienced nurse from Charity's legendary Emergency Room, was another person who was about to see something new and terrifying. "It was such a balmy, windy afternoon, the eye had passed and was heading north, and I could just see us going home that evening. But when we went to sleep that night everything seemed to be changing."[29]

By then, the water surging into the city was growing deeper around Charity. The surge of water came from three directions, the Industrial Canal, the London Canal, and the Orleans Canal. [30]

Later that night John Penland and his wife Mooney Bryant-Penland, an ER nurse, were sleeping in the ER when they were awakened by something out of the *Twilight Zone*. "Look, it's just like in the bathtub, but a whole lot bigger, but I wonder where it's going," John heard a nurse remark. He looked over the edge of the ER ambulance ramp to see a swirling vortex 2 to 3 feet in diameter. Water blasted into the basement quickly through a hole in the exterior wall. They quickly stepped into the ER and looked down the basement stairs to see water rising up the steps. In a few short seconds the entire staff realized the danger of the water flooding the ER.[31]

Everyone—doctors, residents, nurses, aides, security, patients, and cleaning staff—rushed everything upstairs. Beds, monitors, equipment, tables, chairs, everything that was not nailed down swiftly flew up the stairs. [32]

The floodwater was a fatal blow to Charity. It knocked out the elevators, refrigeration system, the cafeteria, the morgue, electrical switching rooms, and destroyed medical records. The pace of the water slowed. It finally halted one step away from the floor of the ER. The great Medical Center of Louisiana was marooned without the very basics of civilization. It would remain in this primitive condition for days.

Charity Hospital would never reopen.

The not so obvious reason that evacuation from the city hospitals was so painstakingly slow is that almost 100,000 residents were in far more precarious situations. They were left exposed at the worst time of the year for insects, heat and humidity on blistering hot asphalt roofs, and many of them had no food, water or sanitation. And many of the very young and very old were weak, ill, and could not stand the extremes of the environment they were forced to endure. To the desperate people clinging for their lives, the hospitals seemed like an oasis—with or without power.

New Orleans was chin-deep in a crisis seen by few other cities in America. Mayor Ray Nagin and Gov. Kathleen Blanco had failed to move decisively. The Regional Transit Authority.'s lack of action to move their buses lost the entire fleet. Hospitals did not expect the sudden calamity they faced.

Stranded Charity doctors and nurses were furious as they hand bagged patients with limited supplies and no word when they would be rescued.

Nearby, Tulane. airlifted their staff out of the flooded hospital.

CNN's Dr. Sanjay Gupta somehow made his way to Charity and filed a gruesome report. "There's no electricity, no running water, no lights. So this is what Charity Hospital looks like in the middle of a natural disaster."[33]

As he paused, the camera panned the auditorium transformed into an ER when the floodwaters had suddenly risen from the basement. "We are in downtown New Orleans," Gupta reported. "This is actually an auditorium that we're standing in now. At one time, it held up to 40 patients all around this place. Several patients still remain here, as well."[34]

Dr. Gupta continued in shocked, solemn tones, "But this is the United States. Tuesday, the governor said this place would be evacuated. Three days later, we watch as medical personnel of Tulane, right across the street, were picked up by helicopters, while Charity's patients, some on ventilators being worked by hand pumps, waited in this parking garage. Last night, this hospital had a good night because nobody died. Fortunate because the morgue, which is in the basement, is flooded. The dead have to wait in the stairwell."[35]

Dr. Gupta had no way of knowing how long the ordeal facing healthcare workers would last. While they sweated and waited for rescue, the nurses earned their Angel wings by staying and caring for their patients. In the following chapters, some of these heroic nurses tell their stories of survival and determination to leave no patient to die alone. And how an army of angels lifted them in the worst moments of the nurses' lives.

Chapter 3

Veterans Health Care
Was Ready for Anything

✕✕✕✕✕

Nothing was going right for Chris Cahill.

The worst storm in the history of the US was about to pounce on his emergency room at the VA Medical Center. The worst manmade disaster in the city's history would be sending floodwaters rising up the sides of the hospital. The National Guard would tell him the hospital could not be rescued quickly. And when the beleaguered refugees could be rescued, the Guard would tell him who and what went first. The hospital had over 700 patients and staff, no power, no elevators in a 12-story building, and medical services would be spotty.

His reaction? He threw a week's worth of clothes, two dogs, and his pirogue in his pick-up and headed for the VA early. Chris is not a shrinking violet nurse. He knows how to command people and assets in a crisis and he is perfectly comfortable in the swirling maelstrom of chaos that was the aftermath of Hurricane Katrina. The complications of both the storm and levee failure presented the medical system with the ultimate challenge. He was up to it.

✕✕✕✕✕

"I was at the hospital on Saturday but not much was happening. I came in due to the impending storm and the fact that I was the director of the Emergency Room (ER) and I felt responsible. I went home to sleep on Saturday night. Not many of the staff in the emergency room believed in the severity of the storm. I kept telling them: 'let's get ready. I'll be here tomorrow morning bright and early. We have a lot to prepare.' I slept at home since I had already evacuated my family,." he said. The next day Chris brought his two dogs, Lou and Scrappy to stay with him at the hospital, as he always did for storms.

Chris's brother was president of the West Jefferson Levee District. The brothers talked with their buddies about the storm: what their plan was, what his plan was, and what Chris's plan was. "My brother knew how serious the storm was," said Chris. "He was very nervous, and he got me in the mood where I was anxious. I am glad to be anxious when I need to be."

The next morning Chris packed his pick-up. He was a trained disaster planner—and a camper. "I packed all my stuff." he said. "I had gallons of water and a pirogue [Cajun canoe] in the back of my truck as well as clothes for the week. I figured we would be there for at least three days according to our plan. I know that things never go as planned, especially in a disaster, so I planned for a little bit longer."

"As I pulled into the hospital, the chief of security said, 'Hey, what are you doing with the boat?'

"Well, you know," I said, "I'm thinking about paddling the boat home." He laughed and said, "'I'll say—you are so crazy!'"

✖✖✖✖✖

For Katrina, the VA Center relied on volunteers. Most of the hospitals had one of two different plans. One plan relied on the regular schedule. The second plan divided the staff into two different teams: an Activation Team and a Recovery Team. This time, VA managers asked for volunteers for the hurricane team. Volunteers are preferred because they are empowered and will usually be more effective. This was an excellent example of the nursing process, proactive steps at their best, and a template for future staffing at the VA.

"It turned out that we had more volunteers than we needed," said Chris. "I had made sure that everybody that Sunday was either leaving or that they were coming in so that we had the right team in place and no extra people. And although we told people that only family members could come with them, no matter who came with them, we allowed them in. We also had a special place for animals," he said.

On Sunday evening, Chris started going through the different units such as ICU, SICU, step down unit, Medical Surgical units, rehab units, and the ER. He recalls: "we had meetings between the managers every so many hours." He thought it was important to describe what they would do if certain things happened. "We considered what would be done if water was an issue," said Chris, "or if windows broke. We also considered what to do if there needed to be any evacuation of any part of the hospital."

On Monday morning, Hurricane Katrina hit Buras, Louisiana, and roared north into New Orleans. Prior to the storm hitting, Chris and his staff moved patients into the hallway in case the windows broke. "We all had our extra lighting and extension cords distributed around," Chris said. "The windows of the Surgical Intensive Care Unit (SICU) were blowing out so we moved all patients from the SICU to the step down unit. The walls in the ER were shaking so we moved all the patients to the urgent care clinic."

Katrina came ashore about 60 miles south of New Orleans preceded by 175 mph winds and a 22 foot storm surge. Even though Buras was an hour's drive south of New Orleans, the outer bands of wind, rain and tornadoes thrashed and pummeled the city for hours. The storm's assault exposed any weakness of every structure it touched. Modern buildings were no safer than old wooden houses. Many of the older houses in the city simply collapsed upon themselves. Many new buildings had the exteriors torn away and many of the windows were smashed to the point of leaking.

Chris grew up in a family whose father was a contractor, which gave him insight into problems he could expect with the construction of the hospital. His premonition proved correct. Windows blew out and walls leaked.. Suddenly, all the patients in Urgent Care had to be moved into a safer location Modern construction was not simply safety insurance from Mother Nature

For a moment, after the water drained out from the flooded streets, Chris thought he would be going home that afternoon. The VA Medical Center was only one block away from the Superdome in a cluster of office buildings. Drainage was a city service that was taken for granted, yet even a heavy rain could make neighborhood streets impassable.

Floodwater churned higher again. Then the hospital lost power from Entergy, and the emergency generators switched on. The center did not have enough emergency generator power to maintain air conditioning, elevators, and laboratories. The hospital turned into an oven that never cooled off.

The heat affected humans and the health technology they relied on. Laboratory machines were designed to function in narrow temperature ranges. Once the temperature rose, the machines could not produce accurate test results. The loss of power knocked out X-ray machines, dialysis machines, machines used to clean surgical instruments. The hospital was crippled by failed elevators. Patients on the upper floors were stuck. Moving them could prove to be difficult.

"We did our best to secure patients as the storm roared through the city," said Chris. "Then the storm was gone. There was some flooding in the streets. However, it was a foot and a half, maybe two feet of water. By then it was Monday mid-morning, and I could project driving my truck home pretty soon. However, by afternoon the water started to rise again, and it was not safe to leave. The VA building lost power during the storm, but generators kept running. The generators lighted the ER, hallways, and the stairwells, but there was no air conditioning. Nurses who were experienced with hurricanes knew what was about to happen in the VA," he said.

"It got hot pretty quickly, and it was just Monday afternoon," said Chris. "The water was coming up fairly fast. We were still doing okay with the patients. The thing we were worried about was the elevator, because we had water come into the SICU, and it went down through the elevators. Staff cleaned up the mess when the water came through the roof in the ER and started to move people back into the emergency room and out of the urgent care area because the lighting was better. We decided to move all the critical care patients down to the ER so we could evacuate them first." said Chris. "So that's what we did. It was a good thing we did because it wasn't long before we lost our elevators, and 14 ventilator patients were in the ER, and the hospital was on emergency power."

Chris was worried that the emergency power might fail. "I told the engineers that I didn't think one generator was enough. I asked them if we had more generators as the water was still rising. They said there were more generators and I said, 'Bring them on!' We put all the generators we had on the emergency room ramp with a barrel of diesel fuel. I've always had fishing camps so I know how to work these things and know what to do. I told the engineers that I also wanted extension cords to all of the ventilator patients so that if my emergency generators went down, I had back-up generators I could crank up, and I wouldn't have to bag the patients. ["To bag" is the term nurses use for ventilating a patient by hand.] And that is just what happened.

Early Tuesday morning, Chris was sleeping in the chief of staff's area and one of the nurses banged on the door. Chris was in his underwear. The nurse was yelling for him to hurry to the emergency room. The staff had just noticed that the water was rising, and they were afraid. The phones were not working.

Ventilator patients had been brought to Chris's unit earlier that night and they now had a total of 17 patients on vents. On initial assessment, their vital signs looked good. "I couldn't do any X-rays or blood gases." said Chris. The X-rays and blood gases were basic diagnostic tools to determine the condition of patients on vents, and without them, the doctors turned to other equipment that worked. "The EKGs looked good so we just took them up, triaged them and took care of them without knowing the history on them.

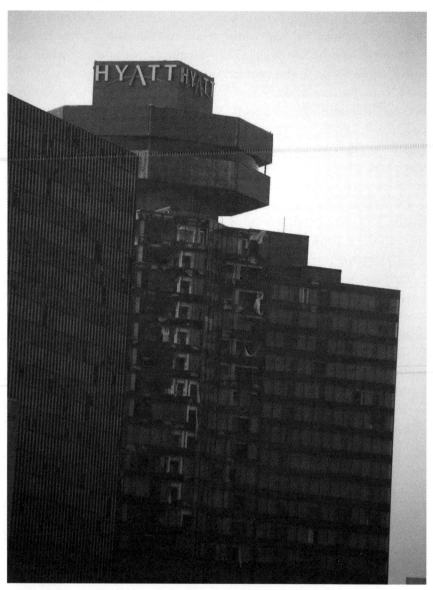

When the New Orleans Police Department lost offices and equipment, the Hyatt Hotel became a temporary command post.

"We gave them the help we could."

When the Louisiana National Guard had lost most of their rescue vehicles in the initial onslaught of Katrina, and made it clear they could not evacuate the hospital immediately, Chris said, "I felt it was unacceptable, and the chief of staff thought so too. So we made the decision to evacuate on our own." The VA had an advantage no other hospital enjoyed: large trucks with high wheel clearance that could run in the rising water and that could be used for evacuating the patients. VA staff drove the trucks from the storage area about 12 miles away on Airline Highway. They took patients to the Superdome. Chris and the other nurses stayed with those patients until they were airlifted out and then communicated with the military that they had 15 more ventilator patients to be evacuated.

"They agreed to airlift them out on their terms." said Chris.

"They would tell us when they were ready for them. And halfway through the day, half of them were airlifted out."

Unfortunately, the remaining ventilator patients could not be moved because the helicopters couldn't fly at night.

There had been reports of shooting at night. No one seemed to know who was shooting or at what. "If you went outside at night, you would hear different types of guns. You could hear little handguns and shotguns, and you could hear what sounded more like military fire. It was only a few helicopters that were flying at night, because they had large spotlights. During the day, if you looked up into the air you would see 10 to 15 helicopters at any point in the day, but at night only one or two," he recalled.

※※※※※

Sometimes the rescuers and Good Samaritans caused flooding problems at the Veterans Center: boat wakes.

"They had to constantly watch the water line as they evacuated the ventilator patients. One of the major problems we had was that the water line rose to within six inches of becoming a problem.

Airboats and motorboats were going down the street, sending waves into the generator room. So we had to develop a means of blocking the water so that when the waves would come, it wouldn't splash the electrical cords on our generators," said Chris.

Fortunately, the hospital had enough fuel for generators and enough food for the patients, staff and walk-up or float-in visitors. They lost one cafeteria in the flooded basement, but the other cafeteria was upstairs with enough food.

Although Tuesday seemed to go well for the VA, it brought problems—and improvised solutions. Like every other hospital that was flooded, one of the most efficient and convenient services failed. The elevators went out. Someone was stuck in one elevator. It was no longer safe to use any of the elevators. With the vertical movement compromised, the question of how to evacuate patients became a dilemma for doctors and nurses. Advanced planning and practice came to the rescue.

Chris decided they would stage everything from the ER. "We had power in the ER," he said. "We had lighting. We were close to food. We had people coming into the ER. People swam in, and floated in. We had a total of 93 patients that we took in during the storm. We ended up evacuating a little over 700 people from the VA Medical Center. Outsiders who came to the VA Hospital were not just seeking shelter. Many were sick," he said.

Chris explained that he had purchased what were called "the Evacusleds."

"An Evacusled is like a transfer board with wheels on it that slides under a mattress," Chris said. "You pull straps over somebody and strap them in. Once you do that, you can pull them down the stairs. And whenever I would train somebody, I would always make them pull me because I'm large. To show them how well it worked, I'd let them pull me down the stairs. It's kind of fun—one of the more fun things I teach."

By Wednesday the ventilator patients had been evacuated, and the staff tried to get everyone else out. By this time they had reached the National Guard. The Guard came Wednesday evening, but the evacuation couldn't start immediately. The problem was that the Evacusleds were in the education building.

Chris took responsibility: he donned his HazMat outfit and swam out a short distance to the education building. "It was quite a show," said Chris. "Staff enjoyed that and got pictures of me! We were in three or four feet of water so I could wade through it. When I got to the building, I couldn't get the door open. So, I had to wade back and get a crowbar and a sledgehammer. I ended up smashing down the door to get into the building. When I smashed the door, the water went into the building too, but I was able to get into the education building and get our sleds. Of course, now everybody had forgotten how to use them, so I had to re-teach everybody!"

First Chris and all of the other managers reassessed all of their patients. They had a rating scale and knew how to determine who was the most critical, and the evacuation was to take them out first. Then Chris and a team of other men, along with some women, would sled patients down the stairs. "We started on the eleventh floor, used the Evacusled to bring patients down to the tenth floor, put them in the bed of my truck, and I would drive them down to the first floor. The most critical patients came from the ICU on the fourth, fifth, and sixth floors. It was very hot with no air conditioning, but we focused on the work. I enjoyed the work because it was important. I'm so compulsive; as long as I'm working I'm happy."

✕✕✕✕✕

Training, experience, proactive decisions, and capital assets made a huge difference in protecting patients, staff, and saving lives at the Veterans Healthcare Center. Evacuation training and heavy assets like huge trucks, allowed the VA to evacuate their patients to regional VA hospitals. In addition, the VA hospital system had an extensive national electronic health record system (EHR) that allowed any hospital to see the records of any patient in the national VA medical system.

How the VA Tracks Veterans And Their Health
—The Consolidated Patient Record System helped save lives during Katrina.

—One of the biggest advantages the VA enjoyed over almost all hospitals was the CPRS. The system is used throughout the 152 VA medical centers

—The system was invented in the 1970s by VA doctors for the VA system, then released in 1997 to any hospital in the country. It is the forerunner of modern electronic healthcare records.

—Any VA patient can go to any VA center anywhere in the country and the doctors can see his or her medical record.

❋❋❋❋❋

Chris, as head of the ER and critical care areas, assumed the role of the "go-to-guy" in the successful evacuation of the VA hospital. "I had become a real hot commodity because I knew how to do things other people didn't know how to do. Even before the storm."

Chris had taken on a disaster management role when New Orleans hosted the Super Bowl in 2000. Because it's only a block away from the Superdome, public safety and football event managers wanted the VA to be a first responder. Chris was the only volunteer from the VA. "They sent me to Little Rock, Arkansas, and I was trained by the Department of Defense and the Department of Veterans Affairs on disaster preparation, decontamination, and that type of training," he explained. "I also recognized the chance to get grants in several categories. The director of nurses loved that I was getting items that we would have missed otherwise. The Evacusleds were one example," Chris said.

"It doesn't matter what state you are in. Our division included parts of Texas, Oklahoma, Arkansas, Louisiana, Mississippi, Florida, and Alabama. The Department of Defense assisted us. They would give us 100 patients," said Chris. "For example, our last drill was that Biloxi was getting a hurricane, and Biloxi had 100 patients that needed to be evacuated. The VA sent ten patients to all different hospitals in the division. That got us to learn how to integrate our network so that we depended upon each other. This helped us develop networking skills and know who has what special services and where to send which patients."

"There was an article in the American Journal of Nursing in November 2005 where you will see the Veterans Administration. You will also see the transport planes and the Houston VA nurses taking on patients from the New Orleans VA. Because we had consolidated record systems, you know everything about them. The patient's name, their social, all their medicines, all their history and what we have done in New Orleans."

✕✕✕✕✕

On Wednesday the National Guard came to pick up patients. They brought what Chris called "these really cool trucks. They are used to build bridges so the engine is on the top and the driver can actually sit in water. We sledded our sick patients down to the ER to be held until the National Guard came to get them. It was amazing how well the Evacusled worked," he explained. "A patient who had a spinal fusion on Saturday went from the SICU on the sixth floor down the Evacusled so easily it was just like a ride. They save lives and they made it easy on the staff," he said.

✕✕✕✕✕

Four days of high stress conditions with relentless, steamy August heat, sleep deprivation, survival diet, and uncertain plans of rescue. It had been playing havoc on the bodies and minds of everyone.

The National Guard brought water and MREs [Meals Ready to Eat] on Wednesday, and more patients were evacuated. Fragile dialysis patients were taken out next, and the remaining ICU patients were evacuated by Thursday. Dialysis patients needed power for their machines, water and regular nursing attention.

Chris's voice changed when he spoke about their first loss of a patient. "Thursday we had a death. He was an ICU patient who was on a special drip, and we knew that his death was imminent. He was a 'do not resuscitate' even before the storm came. It was the first death, and it did throw me."

The morgue was on the third floor. The body was in the ER waiting to be carried out. Chris asked the director, "what we would do with him?" The hospital still didn't have elevators, and it is easier to come down the stairs than go up the stairs. The director's response was to take the deceased up to the morgue on the third floor. It was still cool even though the air conditioner wasn't on.

So that is what Chris did. "I got a spine board," he said, "and put him on the spine board as best as I could to carry him up the stairs. That was very tough, but I made it."

At this point the water seemed to slow, but one of the doctors thought it was still coming up.

Chris knew some things from his previous camping experience. "I would keep watching the water rise because when we were camping, we would put a stick in the mud to keep an eye on the water," he pointed out. "I knew that when there was a wave, it pushes the boards up and they sit there. Then the water goes down, you know. You cannot determine it that way." He marked a No Parking sign with a red marker and showed everyone, then explained, "it is like if you go under a bridge, you'll see sticks with feet and how many feet. We kept the sticks and all was okay—except for the wakes."

Lessons Learned at the VA Center
—During Katrina, Veterans managers asked for volunteers among nurses, doctors and healthcare workers. They got more than they needed.

—The hospital allowed families of workers to stay at the hospital.

—The VA Center had four total deaths, who died on transfer.

—The Evacusled helped staff move critical patients who could not walk from high floors.

—Long extension cords from emergency generators to ventilators helped save critical patients who could not breathe on their own.

—The VA had transportation advantages that other hospitals did not have: trucks with high wheel elevation that could evacuate in flooded streets.

—Military helicopter crews and hospital staff argued who should be evacuated first. Guardsmen wanted to take walking patients and hospital staff first. Hospital staff wanted their most critical patients out first—those on ventilators, dialysis machines and recovering from surgery. Guardsmen prevailed. "They had the guns," said Chris Cahill.

Four guys paddling a hot tub: "It was one of my favorite things during the storm to see what things you saw people paddling in. I saw some people, four guys in a hot tub paddling with shovels and two by fours. I saw a guy in a blow-up baby pool. I saw people on doors, on mattresses and other stuff like people swimming in inner tubes. Unfortunately, people were driving around in boats with guns which was very dangerous.

"On Thursday," said Chris, "I got into a fight with the guy from the National Guard. At this point he was nervous about how the evacuation process was going even though I felt good about it. Apparently, the National Guardsman wanted to take ambulatory patients, women and children, and visitors instead of non-ambulatory patients because he could take a lot of them in one load. So the National Guard said they were not taking any of the non-ambulatory patients and he was going to take women and children now. He wanted to take the visitors, because he could take a lot of them in one load.

"I got very upset," he said. "I did kind of blow my top. I told him that these people are sick, that they have been here for five days. They need to go. They were sitting in the bottom of the parking garage, waiting. And you're here and you're telling me you're going to take out only women and healthy people and you want to take my staff?" He said, 'Yes!'"

Chris realized he had to give in. "At this point it was martial law or whatever you want to call it. They had the machine guns."

This was Thursday night, "the roughest night for me. I was now upset that my evacuation plan had been put to the side."

It was almost dark, and the National Guard filled a helicopter with a load of people who could walk. Guardsmen said they would come back for one more load. When Chris asked if they were going to help carry the other remaining patients back upstairs, he reported their answer: "They said: 'Of course not.' They don't do that. When I asked if they were going to help us carry these patients back upstairs, they said: 'Of course not.'"

"They said they don't do that," Chris recalled.

"They just sat there with the guns."

Chris came up with a new plan. He knew that the Guardsmen wouldn't take those patients, he decided to make sure they helped the staff move them from the parking lot back to the main area, the emergency room.

The VA evacuation went more smoothly than any other hospital in South Louisiana. Still, the VA suffered similar problems like every other hospital. The military in charge of evacuation had a priority of patients to be evacuated—and the hospital had quite a different priority. Medical staff members were surprised and angered when the helicopter evacuation teams refused to evacuate medically-fragile patients. They wanted to evacuate ambulatory patients, visitors and nurses instead.

But nurses are accustomed to dealing with challenging personalities that do not improve in a crisis, and they managed the situation by compromise, reason, and more flexible objectives.

Chris explained that when the National Guard returned later that evening they agreed to the new plan. "Staff brought the last of their non-ambulatory patients to the emergency room as well as the last of the wheelchair patients. Instead of evacuating the women and children and staff, they first took all of my ambulatory patients and lined them up and the military did not know who they were. They just knew they were ambulatory and they had their chart. They knew where they were going, and when they got to the staging area on Airline Highway, they were separated there.

"We snuck our patients out without the military's consent." said Chris. They were going to take the nurses and leave us with nobody. Now we did allow some nurses to leave." At that point he sent out the nursing staff who had children. So a child and a patient looked like a little family.

"The next day, Friday, helicopters made three or four more trips and got everybody out, including nurses, the management team, and some of the managers that were not feeling well. They were stressed-out or physically exhausted to the point that I didn't think they were really helping. Most of the managers were getting about three hours of sleep a night it was so hot. All of the VA staff had been working 12-hour shifts for five days," he said.

The VA had four total deaths. They died on transfer. The deaths bothered Chris, because that was the purpose of not moving the critical care patients in the first place. "If other non-VA facilities want to transfer them to our ER or the ICU, we generally say no," he said. "They're critical and they will probably die as they are transported, so we're not going to take a chance they might die enroute. And it is the same concept in a disaster."

✕✕✕✕✕

Finally, on Friday, September 2, Chris left the VA hospital. "I was finished," he said. "I had done my duty and I had done well. They wanted to know where I wanted to go. I had friends in Jackson, Mississippi, so I said I want to go to Jackson, and to Jackson we went." said Chris. "We got about halfway down the street, and I asked the bus driver to please pull over at this gas station. He asked what for?'

"I said, 'I need a beer' and so I actually convinced him to pull over," Chris smiled, "so I ended up getting a bunch of alcohol, and we had a party in the back of the bus, with all my nurses and security and my disaster team. We had a great time. We all drank and slept and talked. I then woke up in Jackson, Mississippi," he said.

"There was a team there waiting to take care of us. They fed us and asked what we wanted to do." Chris wanted to fly to his family. "The first time I talked to my family was probably Thursday sometime. I got a text message first and where they were. I flew to

Atlanta where I had like a three-hour layover in which time I ate McDonald's, Burger King, Wendy's, and TGI Fridays. I wanted to taste a little bit of everything. Even though I was in these pajama scrub-type clothes, I really didn't care." Chris flew from Atlanta to Pensacola, and his family picked him up there.

Chris spent the week in Florida. "There were twenty-plus people in the house, but it was all of my relatives," he said, "so I was okay with that. We returned to New Orleans, to the scene of the crime. Back to New Orleans, back to the emergency room of the VA where everything was staged and by this time we had security, federal police officers, who were guarding buildings because they were afraid of looters."

✖✖✖✖✖

Chris's family owns a grammar school. They began to recover the property. One building was destroyed, but others weren't and Chris and his brothers began working on the school to get it ready." We planned to open the first of October." said Chris.

"However, the director of nursing called me, and told me that there was a need for me at the VA. So I returned to work at the VA to help recover the hospital. I assisted taking care of the security and police personnel, and then I concentrated on setting up the clinics."

VA Awards Chris Cahill the Valor Award

In October 2005, less than a month after Katrina, the Veterans Administration awarded Chris Cahill the Valor Award for Heroic Efforts in risking his life to save the lives of others. Cahill and his wife were flown to the White House where he was presented the honor by the Secretary of Veterans Affairs James Nicholson and an aide to President George W. Bush. Bush had been scheduled to present the award, but had to cancel at the last minute due to an emergency speech. Cahill is the first nurse in VA history to receive the award. And if there is an angel who is playful and devoted to his mortals, let us nominate Chris as his representative at the VA.

Chapter 4

Pendleton Memorial Hospital: Closest to the Eye of Katrina

"There are times when you have a defining moment in life and Hurricane Katrina was one of them," Carol Beck McCullough said. "I saw the best there was in humanity, heroism, and camaraderie."

At first glance, the energetic dark brunette may remind you of a cheerful Italian mother, smiling, looking directly into your eyes. Carol is perfectly relaxed with the responsibilities and demands of a command position. The self-described control freak expects positive results and is willing to work hard to get them. She has always been dedicated to the care of her staff, and they have returned the love with a willingness to meet her demands.

Carol Beck McCullough was the director of nursing at Pendleton Memorial Methodist Hospital when Katrina struck. As director, she was destined to lead her nurses through five days of harrowing crisis after crisis in unbelievably difficult circumstances that would have crushed many other leaders. As critical systems failed throughout the hospital, Carol was the leader who stepped up to guide her staff forward without fear or hesitation.

Pendleton Memorial Methodist Hospital was a six-story hospital in the part of town called New Orleans East. It is one of the newer communities of the city reclaimed from the swamps and bayous that surround New Orleans. It's been known as the development and assembly site for NASA space vehicles. The gleaming white and silver exterior made Pendleton an easily visible landmark.

Pendleton was a full-service, big-city hospital run by an experienced staff. There was a limit to their experience. Only a few of the staff were experienced in surviving a hurricane of unprecedented ferocity that produced a flood of historic magnitude. The structure stood almost directly in the path of the ultimate forces of Hurricane Katrina.

As the director of nursing, Carol faced this challenge, set the example for her nurses, and led them and their patients through hell to survival. As she spoke, the torment and the crisis returned to her. It is only a few short weeks after the disaster and she sees her nurses and patients vividly in her memory. The emotions are overwhelming. We talked, we cried about the incredible events she lived through. This is her story. [1]

※※※※※

"We knew on Friday afternoon prior to Katrina hitting that we would probably have to go into the hospital for the duration," said Carol. "The decision wasn't really made until Saturday because on Friday it still looked like Katrina might go to Apalachicola, Florida. We cut back on elective admissions, elective surgeries and that type of thing. It is very costly when you decide to defend in place. So it is a big decision when you start looking at that cost. It is a huge decision."

During Hurricane Ivan in 2004, Pendleton and Chalmette General Hospital, a sister facility, that was also owned by Universal Health Services of Pennsylvania, were thought to be among the few private hospitals that evacuated patients. Patients were airlifted by helicopter with nursing staff to Lake Charles in Southwest Louisiana, which proved to be expensive. Hospital leadership drew heat for evacuating the critical patients. Further complicating the decision was the fact that for-profit hospitals are not generally reimbursed for such expenses by government health programs.

The erratic nature of the forecasts of Hurricane Katrina prompted last-minute adjustments in planning. The NWS did not predict the storm would come into Louisiana until the 10 p.m. forecast the Friday before the storm.

CEO Larry Graham decided to go fishing, but found an ugly surprise when he returned—Katrina was heading for New Orleans.[2] Saturday, barely 36 hours before the hurricane came ashore,

Carol was consulting with Graham, and the chiefs of the medical staff. Together, they made the decision to go in to the hospital for the storm, and they told everybody it was essential that they be there between 10 a.m. Sunday morning and 4 p.m. that afternoon. The "designated staff" were needed to care for the remaining patients, and certain physicians.

Their ordeal began on Sunday morning, August 28. Carol summoned her managers, the managers called their nurses, and the managers alerted other staff. She discovered the cruel reality that three of her vital nurse managers were missing. One was out-of-state on vacation. Two were only 40 miles away in Mississippi, but they could not get through the contraflow evacuation traffic. Carol called the Louisiana State Police and the National Guard but nothing could be done to help her vital managers get to the

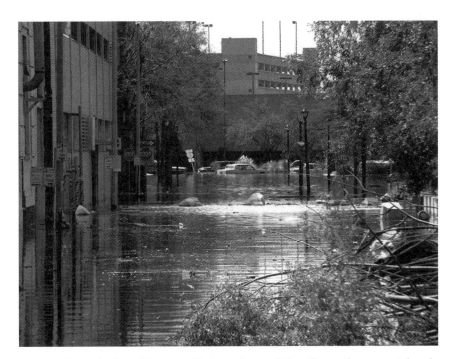

Hospitals including Charity, University and Pendleton became islands surrounded by floodwaters sometimes chest high.

hospital. Mayor Ray Nagin had called for a mandatory evacuation of New Orleans with the exception of hotels and hospitals. Nobody could get into the city. They all wanted out.

Mostly all. About 100,000 stayed behind. Too poor to leave. Too stubborn. Too scared.

"We started trying to get some patients transferred out to safer locations, especially our ventilator patients," said Carol. "We just couldn't find any support or way to transport them out. There was no hospital that would take them because nobody was still really sure where the storm was going to hit. Katrina was such a monster that nobody wanted to take a chance on where it would come ashore. So we couldn't get the patients moved. We were stuck."

Carol had over 100 patients to care for and, including staff and families, a total of 750 people were in the hospital.

Most of the New Orleans-area hospitals routinely allowed essential

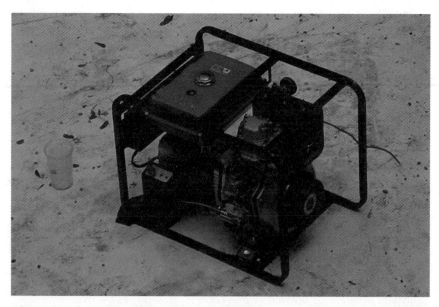

Those people aware of the ugly possibilities prayed for generators. Here is a portable generator used at Charity Hospital that continued working even when huge emergency generators drowned in the basement and ground floor.

personnel, their families and dependents into the hospital during hurricanes. "The families typically had little bitty babies, toddlers, teenagers, crippled grandmothers who lived with them," Carol said. "It was bedlam in some ways, just bedlam." Some hospitals like Ochsner Medical Center, allowed family dogs, cats, and other smaller pets, all of which required at least daily attention.

Carol estimated that 25 house-based and private-practice physicians made it into the hospital, including major specialties: orthopedics, obstetrics, general surgery, vascular surgery, and radiology. Everything the hospital needed was onsite, and all of the clinical services were staffed. She felt confident Pendleton was prepared.

"What we weren't ready for was the fact that we were going to lose power and we would be without power for up to a week," Carol said. Most hospitals with sealed windows are huge consumers of power for air conditioning, refrigeration, and vital medical devices like ventilators, telemetry units, and infusion machines. And without these services, the hospitals quickly become saunas.

"Sunday we got everybody in the hospital that we could find. We had 51 patients who were having their hearts monitored on two units, and we moved all of those patients onto one unit. Staff worked out various scenarios. For example, what were they going to do with the kitchen equipment? What were they going to do about radiology, the lab and all of those services that were on the first floor and likely to be flooded? Staff had planned for such scenarios, but had never had to put those plans into place. They designated areas where the dietary department could be located. They placed some freezers and refrigeration units up on the sixth floor in areas that could be used as a staging area for dietary," she said.

Although Pendleton did not have a water well, drums of water were stored so they had extra water for flushing and for bathing strategically placed around the hospital. "We also had spent the majority of my time figuring out who's here. How many are we sleeping? Who needs to sleep with whom? I've got nurse A with her husband and two kids and nurse B with her six kids. As we went around we tried to figure out how many beds we could put into these various rooms and how many cots we could place. That took up an easy eight hours," she said, "just making sure I had some place for everybody to bed down. Once you get them a spot and you get them sheets, they can bed down, they're fine. When the kids are settled, then people tend to settle down, and things go a lot smoother. With everybody milling around, it was just too chaotic. I didn't know who was there. I couldn't keep up with what was going on. I'm a control freak, and I can't tolerate chaos."

The controlling part of her character was about to meet its worst nightmare.

As Katrina approached shore on Monday, the outer feeder bands of heavy rain howled and hurled rain at the hospital at almost 200 miles per hour. In the darkness of the early morning hours, the rain was coming in so hard that it pierced the sealed windows, and ran into Carol's office. Water ran down the walls of her office. "I was sleeping okay until the building started to leak, my feet were wet, and I took a few minutes to wake up because I was so exhausted." She quickly moved her belongings to an office nearby to stay dry. The hurricane force winds were only a hint of disaster.

Wind unpeeled the heating and air conditioning vents on top of the building, leaving an entrance for water to pour in on the sixth-floor patients. Carol had to start moving all of the people sleeping in empty rooms on the sixth floor, along with the patients who were on six and two nursing units. This meant she had to wake people up. Telling them she was sorry, she said, "I've got to have this room. I know I gave it to you, but now you can't have it. And please, you've got to hurry up because we've got to move patients. The water is coming in, and you have to move."

Carol shook her head ruefully. "Nobody was happy at that point in time. I don't think there was a happy soul in the entire building. And as fast as we moved people from one room, another vent would blow away. It was like the Keystone cops! We were pushing beds around. I was running around sweating like a pig, but I got everybody settled again."

Soon vents disappeared off on the other side of sixth floor over the long-term care unit. This area was a hospital-within-a-hospital where many of the patients died. They were extremely frail, mostly elderly individuals. Rooms had to be found quickly for them because filthy water was coming off the roof through the ceiling and the vents.

Just as soon as one crisis abated, another followed.

"The wind was howling, but the building was standing," Carol said. Then the hospital lost windows. Huge windows began imploding. "Glass was flying everywhere into the building," said Carol. "The medical surgical units had a huge bank of windows in the nurses station and I had just bunches of people on that unit. And when the window went out, the first thing you worried about is 'who got hurt?' And by the grace of God, nobody got hurt when the windows went. Someone could have been killed."

Staff had set up children's play areas on those units because the spaces were light and airy looking. Many people with big families had been put there to sleep because there was room for their kids to move around so they wouldn't feel cramped. "And then there go the windows again," said Carol. "We did have some minor injuries that just scared the living you know what out of everybody during this exploding glass window terror. I was terrified that somebody was going to be seriously hurt."

"I was down at the emergency room talking to my folks. Most of the people, like the folks in the ER, bedded down in the ER because until after the storm is passed, they would not get any business in the ER. Nobody travels, nobody's driving to come to the ER so they bedded down there and they had their kids and their families down there in the treatment room."

Carol and her staff were trying to secure the ambulance bay doors because the wind was still gusting through. "I was standing there trying to figure out how we're going to secure the doors," Carol recalled, "and looking out on the parking lot, and I felt water coming in.

"I said, 'Guys, get your patients, get them on the stretchers, and get out of here.'

"They said 'what are you talking about?'"

"You see that water? It's come up three inches since I've been standing here"

"'Oh that's just rainwater,' they said."

"Oh, no! See, I think the lake has overtopped the levee."

Pendleton was only several hundred feet from 660 square-mile Lake Pontchartrain, and the team feared they would be flooded from the lake water being blown over the levee. It was a scenario they had heard about in years past. Now it came true.

"The director of the ER, whose car was parked right outside the entrance to the ER, said, 'Oh my goodness, it's up to midway on my tires.'"

"Guys, get your stuff. Let's go! Move! Move now!"

"It was no time then until the water hit the generator," Carol said. The generator was on the ground floor, about four feet off the ground, and it lost power. They still had power in the tower because the tower generators were on the roof. The pump that drives the diesel fuel to the roof was on the ground. Eventually it failed.

Ironically, the city and state building code may have required generators. Codes made no specific mention that the generators should be located above the flood plain, as should electrical switching equipment and fuel storage. Like all of the other hospital generators in South Louisiana, Pendleton's were doomed to fail. But for a precious few hours the tower generator continued operating, allowing air conditioning and ventilators to function. The hospital could breathe.

The working generator provided the hospital a few hours of air conditioning and power that was rare at other local hospitals. "The labor and delivery area was in the tower and we had women in labor. Then we moved babies out of the nursery and put them in the tower because those babies had no temperature of their own, so we had to maintain their temperature. The major cardiac catheter laboratory was there, as were the outpatient laboratories. Staff were able to move patients into the tower because they still had central air conditioning in that area. "We figured that these people are just so fragile," said Carol, "that we wanted to try to do something with them."

✳✳✳✳✳

In a second bit of good luck, the Pendleton seemed secure in one sense. About 150 National Guardsmen and police officers were camped on the sixth floor. News and rumors spread throughout the New Orleans area of looting and lawlessness—even snipers—downtown. The staff was comforted to have the guardsmen and policemen.

At that point they were still able to use mobile phones and sometimes could use land lines.

As Monday night approached, the rising water and uncertainty of evacuation forced a retreat of supplies and medical equipment to the second floor. Dietary, pharmacy, laboratory equipment, and material that were still serviceable from central supply were all moved. Batteries and flashlights, two valuable commodities when the lights go out, appeared to be adequate. "We thought we had enough, but when you've got 750 people in the building, without lights, then those flashlights and batteries don't last very long," she said.

Tuesday morning the situation looked relatively stable for Pendleton. Generators were working in the tower allowing some comfort for 29 patients in ICU, the labor and delivery patients, and the newborns. Carol seized the moment to support her staff by checking on them and showing a visible presence of her leadership.

"I spent most of Tuesday," she said, "just walking around, making sure that everyone had a place to sleep. I was out there so people could see what was going on and trying to make sure that my nurses were hanging in. I wanted to be sure that they were getting sleep. We were on 12- hour shifts. I also made sure people didn't mess with them when they were trying to sleep because I needed them desperately."

"Things were happening with the other administrators too. On Monday afternoon the CEO had to go to surgery. He had an infection that had developed from something on his right buttocks. It was really bothering him. I asked the doctors to call the surgeon right away. They had to lance it, drain it, and pack it. He was put on IV antibiotics, and put on the sofa in his office to recover from general anesthesia and surgery. He was pretty well out of it," she said.

Although Tuesday got off to a relatively positive start, Pendleton started to deteriorate.

Four to five feet of filthy flood water surrounding the hospital appeared to be rising once more. Toilets started backing up because there was no water pressure, and they had no running water with 750 people in the building. Finally the last generators failed and power failed. The nurses were forced to manually "hand-bag" the 14 patients on ventilators to help them breathe.

"At that point, we realized we had nothing. We did not have water. We did not have sanitation. We had no power, no generator—we had nothing. By Wednesday it was probably close to 115 degrees in the building. I had nurses giving nursing care with IVs running into their arms because they were so dehydrated. We had water, but we were trying to stretch it," she said.

"The flood outside wasn't going down and we did not know how long we were going to be there. So we were rationing drinking water. Some people have a lower tolerance for water intake than other people do. And it was so hot. When the heat started, people started losing it."

Surrounded by conditions intolerable in any hospital, Carol knew she had to remain a symbol of inspiration to her staff.

It was the ultimate test of a person and a nurse leader.

"I knew I couldn't lose it. You had to reach down inside of yourself, and pull it from your toes. And when I'd feel like I was getting ready to lose it, I would just disappear for a few minutes until I could get myself back together again. I didn't know where my husband was. I didn't know how to get in touch with them. No cell phones were working, and the land lines were out. Nobody had any kind of communication."

By late Tuesday afternoon the wind was gone. Water was about five feet deep in the parking lot. Carol could barely see the top of her Jeep. Debris was floating all around the hospital.

"There were alligators swimming in the water," she said. "There were snakes. We hoped they stayed outside."

On Tuesday night, Carol heard a loud roar. She couldn't figure out what it could be. It was the water going down the elevator shaft into the basement. "It sounded like Niagara Falls," she said. "It was just an awful noise." Carol didn't remember being scared. "I remember being really upset about the nurses and the patients. I remember being worried about my husband. And I remember thinking that my father is going to be going bananas because he wouldn't know what was happening with me."

"My dad is almost 82 but he's very active. He was in his RV coming back from California with his girlfriend. I knew he was somewhere in the middle of the country but wasn't quite sure where. I had a cell phone number for him, but that didn't do any good. Sometime, I think it was Wednesday morning; I was able to get through on a cell phone to my brother on his landline and let him know that I was okay. I asked him to get in touch with Daddy to let him know. I gave him my husband's cell phone number and asked them to contact my husband also to let him know that I'm all right.

"Sometime Tuesday, one of the Pendleton maintenance staff members went out in a boat that he had brought with a husband of one of the doctors. They went out in the boat and stole some diesel fuel. And they had it in drums. Those guys went in the horrific water, got in the boat, and then came back. They unloaded the diesel and muscled that big drum up six flights of stairs in the ungodly heat. They worked on top of the roof, trying to get that generator primed without having a pump.

"If there is sainthood anywhere, that man deserves it. He saved those patients' lives. He was able to get the generator going! We didn't have AC airpower anywhere except labor and delivery. We had emergency power in ICU. With generator power, staff could run the ventilators, and could take care of the babies that were delivered," she said.

"It was just like a miracle," said Carol. "He performed an absolute miracle. If it hadn't been for him, we would've lost them all. As it was, we did lose some. We had to bag the patients for about 12 hours." The nurses kept switching off as one person could only hand-bag a patient for 20 to 30 minutes at a time. "We couldn't do anything for dialysis patients," said Carol. "A patient can't have dialysis without running water."

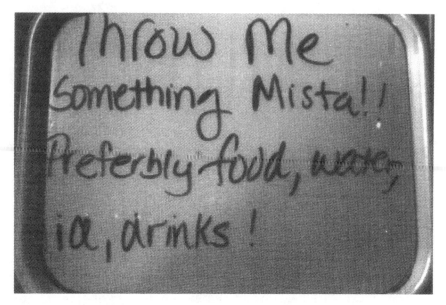

A food tray at Charity Hospital has simple requests.

"Food was not plentiful but we had some. It wasn't the best, but we had it. Dietary thawed out the rolled turkey breast and cold vegetable soup, and huge cans of fruit cocktail. The mothers bought formulas for their babies, but they had not planned on being there that long. Around Wednesday afternoon we were starting to run out of baby formula. So we hit the nursery, and got all of the samples of formula we needed. Then we went to central supply and got all the specialty formula we had, and passed that out to the moms. They were out of diapers. We only had newborn size because we didn't have a pediatric unit, and we didn't have toddler size. So they were putting two newborn sizes together, and that was fine."

In a region where mass communications had crashed, rumors were rampant and the national media reporters covering the event were guilty of reporting inaccurate stories. One of the worst stories concerned the hospitals on the East Bank of the Mississippi River in New Orleans. On more than one occasion hospital staff sitting in marooned hospitals were surprised to hear media report their hospitals had been evacuated.

Carol learned of a report that Pendleton had been evacuated. She knew it was wrong.

"That is when I really got scared. And we felt like, you know, people just forgot we were here. You heard the radio talking about Memorial Baptist, about East Jefferson, about Ochsner, and they talked about all those other hospitals. And nobody—nobody— mentioned Pendleton. I had people and patients at the Lakewood facility—our sister campus—that we couldn't contact. We had no idea what was going on with them. And they were a smaller building. They were only three stories. We had no idea what was going on with them because, we had no way to communicate and no way to get there."

Sometime Wednesday, Carol and other staff members were sitting in administration offices, still trying to keep track of everything and trying to keep some records. "I was without sleep and just kind of walleyed by this time. I had never been that long without a shower in my life. Suddenly this guy walks in, and he's wet from the waist down and he's somebody that we didn't know." Carol described the sudden arrival.

"This guy came in, and he walks to my CEO and says, 'Larry Graham, I presume.' My CEO says, 'Yes.' It was like something out of a movie. He says, 'I'm Jim and I'm from corporate. Our company sent down 18-wheelers with diesel and supplies, and they were staged over on I-10. The problem was that FEMA confiscated them. Our company sent boats and helicopters, and FEMA confiscated them."

FEMA had said they couldn't get to Pendleton but "Jim from corporate" came without even knowing the area. "He got a boat, came across the lake and got them to let him out at the levee on Hayne Boulevard," Carol recalled. "He came over the railroad tracks, over the levee, and waded up Read Boulevard to our hospital. But FEMA couldn't get to me?"

Carol did not mince words when she talked.

"FEMA should rot in hell. It would be a real good thing if I never see Michael Chertoff or Michael Brown in my entire lifetime again. I would probably spit in their face. My patients would not have died if they had done their damn jobs. I am so angry. I get so angry every time I think about it. Brown was sitting there worried about what color of damn shirt he's going to wear, and my patients were dying!"

"Anyway," Carol went on, "this guy is so funny. He says, 'Larry Graham, I presume? I'm from corporate. I was sent to help you.' So what could he do, then, after he had all the trouble getting here? It was just hilarious. Bless his heart for coming. He had one of those—I'm not sure what to call them—but it was one of those super-duper cell phone things that had some kind of really super-duper signal or whatever. And so we were able to call out using his phone. What Jim had was a satellite phone. And we could get out sometimes. It was really good. But the CEO could call corporate and have corporate try to get somebody to come and get us. And let them know what dire straits we were in."

By Wednesday the shortage of food and supplies was acute.

The miracle maintenance man rose to the occasion. He and his guys went out to the medical office building in front of the hospital. They broke in. They went through all the offices looking for bottled water and any food they could find. A couple of the nurse managers, including Carol, had pass keys to all the offices. They went to everybody's desks and got all of the granola bars and candy—whatever they could find—and brought it all back.

"When the maintenance guys went over there and broke in the building, they found this little bitty old lady who was the cutest thing you ever saw in your life. She was a little African-American lady, skinny as a rail, gray hair all done up on her head. She was as neat as a pin, sitting there in the lobby of the medical office building."

No one had any idea how she got into the building. Carol thought she had probably been there for three or four days.

She was just sitting there waiting for somebody to come get her.

"She was in her late 80s early 90s," said Carol "just cute as a bug. We brought her in. The emergency room guys had set up the ER in the outpatient surgery area on the second floor. So I went in there to see about her. They had taken her history, and her blood pressure was low, she was dehydrated and she was hungry. By the time I got down there, she was eating cold vegetable soup and carrying on a conversation, just as bright as you please. She was just the cutest thing you'd ever want to see!"

The lack of air conditioning, the rationing of food and water, and a sense of abandonment haunted many of the hospital staff, patients and a growing number of people who walked up or waded in.

All through the disaster people from the neighborhood just kept coming into the hospital. "More people had kept coming in, coming in, coming in. We had to let them in as there was no place for them to go. We had some guys that were starting to get a little bit horsey. They were fussing and making accusations that the staff was getting better than they were getting. And these people were from the community."

Carol reacted to their complaints. "Hey, I told one of them—by this point in time I was over it. I was really way over it. I said: 'you don't like the accommodations, you know where door is. Knock yourself out! There will be absolutely no problem. Nobody will try to stop you!' And I meant it! I was beyond caring whether or not someone liked the accommodations! I was way beyond that!"

✕✕✕✕✕

The first patients they wanted to move were the mothers and babies, because they were frightened for the babies. Nurses were also worried about families that had very young babies and children. They got together and decided that anybody that had children under the age of two needed to be evacuated. "As they were all able to walk, we thought they would be picked up first," she said.

"We thought we had it all arranged," said Carol, "but when the helicopters would land, they would say no we're not going to take that kind of patient, they were going to take this kind of patient."

Helicopter crews refused to take the critical patients. Many wanted only to take those patients who could walk. Carol said, "It seemed to depend on the kind of helicopter, where they were going, and once they left this, we had no control over their destination." All the patients' medications, the charts, chargebacks, everything was put in a plastic bag and put with the patient for evacuation. And then the patient was taken up to the roof to wait for the next helicopter.

"By now the sanitation situation was so terrible no one had ever seen anything like it," said Carol. "People were using the bathrooms, but by this time they were putting plastic bags in the wastebaskets, and then tying them in a bag. "It was the best you could do," said Carol. Nurses had gone into the wound center and gotten all of the alcohol wipes. They had gone in all the patient rooms, and brought out all the alcohol and hand sanitizer. They retrieved all of the baby wipes from the nursery and from central supply so that people could at least cleanse with them. After the maintenance men went out in the water, Carol recalled, "they would practically bathe with the wipes and that hand sanitizer."

Patients had to be carried up several flights to the roof by hand because there was no electricity to run the elevators. The ones who were real challenges were gastric bypass patients, two of whom weighed over 500 pounds.

"We used ten guys with sheets to carry the patients up the stairs," said Carol. "It was unbelievable, they just muscled them upstairs." Carol remembered one female bypass patient, whose surgery had been done the Friday before the storm, "And normally they go home," she said. "She would've gone home Monday or Tuesday at the latest. She had no complications but she was refusing to walk. She was whining like a baby and refusing get up out of bed." Carol lost her patience.

"Finally, I told her, 'Do you want die?' I said, 'Because if you do want to die, you keep this up! If you want to live, get your feet on the floor and come on. Otherwise, I'm not carrying you. You will walk or you will die.' I had never talked to a patient like that in my life —and God willing, I never will again."

"These guys, my men, were just on their last legs," Carol said. "I mean they could not physically do anymore. And, you could only push people so far and then they just collapsed. And we could not afford for these guys to collapse on us. We needed them so badly.

And for her to just be doing her little baby whiny thing was more than I could handle right then. But she got up. Son of a gun! Picked up her bed and walked! It worked, off she went. She was slow, and she bitched the whole time, but she went."

The Pendleton staff managed to get all the patients upstairs, even those in bad shape. "We had one that was all contracted. It was just pitiful," said Carol.

"Pitiful, pitiful, pitiful. We got him up on the roof, and then the helicopter decided they were not going to take that patient. Well, do you take them back downstairs or do you leave them up there and cover them up?" When the helicopters came down, it generated a horrific wind. Carol said, "I was taking roof material, that gravelly stuff that they put on top of roofs, out of my hair for over a week and a half." Off and on all Wednesday night, the exhausted nurses sent people off the roof until, about 3 or 4 a.m. the helicopters stopped flying.

At last Carol went downstairs to her room and lay down.

Carol's rest didn't last long. "I'll never forget this. I couldn't have been down more than twenty minutes, and I mean, I just passed out," she said. "When I lay down I just passed out cold. I was in filthy scrubs by now, but I didn't care. We had cut the legs off. I had a part of the leg tied into a headband, and oh I was beautiful."

Carol's COO and one of the other nurses came to her room "and tried to talk to me to get up, and I just wasn't even moving. The COO nudged her foot with his foot. "I jumped twenty feet," said Carol, "and screamed bloody murder. He said it took ten years off his life, scared him to death. I had been in that first phase of a deep sleep. I was just totally unconscious to the world because I was so tired. So I had about thirty minutes of good sleep, then, and that was the first rest in 24 hours. But helicopters were coming back again, so everyone had to get up and go."

So Carol climbed back up upstairs, and she and the others kept going that whole Thursday.

"Thursday night, I think I lay down on a cot up on top the roof for about 15 minutes and it was very cold there. I guess because at that point in time with the adrenaline flowing and everything, I was freezing to death. I was so cold. The wind came up and I don't know why, but I was shivering. I lay down there, and I think I slept maybe 20 minutes I woke up and started helping organize patients and moving them up to the roof. I was carrying people, walking people. It was okay that there was no rest. It was okay."

Thursday had been a day of hope for many people stranded in hospitals in New Orleans. It was a day of helicopters, flying, and fleeing the flooded hospitals for destinations out by bus to Baton Rouge, North Louisiana, Houston. Although many thought their ordeal was over and a return to civilization was imminent, some were surprised to find out that the situation was only growing more complicated, and there was a distinct possibility it could grow much worse. Friday was not the day that many people expected.

"We warned everybody. 'Do not get on the military helicopters,'" said Carol. Tenet Healthcare had sent some helicopters, and we had private helicopters that we could control where they were going. We had set up arrangements with North Shore hospital at Slidell, only 15 miles north, that we could stage our staff from there. They had made arrangements with one of our flight facilities in Dallas. It was as close as they could get to us because everything was full of patients and staff. Where were they going to take us? The flight facility had a new addition that did not have patients yet. So that's where they were going to take us. And they were ready for us. They were waiting on us.

Some folks, said Carol "were going to get on whatever helicopter landed. Some of them ended up on I-10 in Metairie. And some of them ended up in the airport. And you can flip a dime over which one of those was worst. Some of the earlier folks who were evacuated ended up at the Superdome. And that's what we were afraid would happen to our staff. That's why we were telling them don't go with the military, because we knew that once the helicopter lifted off, we had no way of knowing where they would land."

"I was on the second-to-last helicopter that left and I went to the Northshore. This was midday on Friday. And man, I didn't care what it cost or what I had to pay. I had to have a shower! I'll go in a patient room. I don't care, just give me a hose! So I got a shower and changed clothes. And they fed us. Some of our people were able to get showers. Then we got on the buses for Dallas. We got to Dallas early, still dark on Saturday morning. We had traveled all night too. There were two buses in the contingent that I was on, and there was a second contingent coming behind us that left later that day.

"Once I got all of our folks in bed, I called the Dallas Hyatt. I said, 'Give me a room. I want a room, I don't care what it costs, and I want it.' And I got a room. I gave my number to the people there at the flight facility. I said, 'My people need me, this is where they can find me–at the Hyatt and this is the number.'"

"The first thing I did was shower, and I ran the water as hot as I could run it. I stayed in there up until I turned into a prune. And I got into those clean sheets, and I cranked that air conditioner way down as low as it could go. I got up late Saturday afternoon and went downstairs. I forgot how much I had to drink. I don't even remember how much, but I drank a lot. I drank a lot.

"I returned to my room went back to bed again. I got up Sunday morning, found a church, and I went to church. They were the nicest people. Somehow or another, they realized I was a refugee. I had no idea how they knew that, but it was possible because I was in jeans and tennis shoes in one of the nicer churches around. And it was so nice. One of the ladies took me to the mall because I needed to get some clothes. I really wanted to put on something decent. I went to the mall and that was the sweetest thing. And I did some shopping. I was able to find the Vodafone store and get a charger. The charger to my phone was lost. I have no idea where it went and it was completely dead. I was able to get in touch with my dad and my brother and my best friend. She lives in Jacksonville and was panic-stricken because she is a nurse and they heard all the horror stories. She knew I would be there at the hospital.

"I flew out of Dallas that Thursday, but my husband didn't want me to come back here because he had not been back to the house yet. We had no idea what condition the house was in. He was in a place in Baton Rouge staying with his eldest daughter, his ex-wife, and the boyfriend in the boyfriend's mother's home in Baton Rouge. He didn't want to come back here until we figured out whether I had anything to come back to. So he and his daughter went down there, and they had to cut trees to get there. I came back ten days after Katrina hit. I flew on to Baton Rouge, was picked up there and brought home.

"My dad was in Kansas and Nebraska when Katrina hit. He stayed put because he figured we were going to be in trouble. And I was able to tell my brother get in touch with dad and tell them that I might need the RV. So that's what my dad did. He brought us that RV. We parked it in my nephew's front yard. He lives in Covington and they had power. We had no power at our house. We also had no water. So we stayed our nephew's front yard for almost two weeks, while we worked on our house we were finally able to get power. We had a generator but it went underwater. We got about five feet of water under the house. We had two big trees that had fallen and hit the roof but no water in the house. The house is over eight feet off the ground so we were very lucky."

Lessons Learned

—Most of the hospital administrators interviewed by the congressional report on Katrina cited time and money as the two most important factors in evacuations.

—Pendleton CEO Larry Graham testified that by the time it was obvious that Katrina would hit the city, it was too late to move patients. The cost of evacuating patients for private, for-profit hospitals was not reimbursed by FEMA.

—Pendleton Hospital staff distrusted some National Guard and Coast Guard helicopter crews because they did not know where the evacuees would be taken. Some refused to evacuate the most critical patients and chose patients able to walk.

—Gastric bypass patients, two weighing over 500 pounds, had to be carried to the roof for evacuation by helicopter.

—Pendleton's ground floor emergency generator, soon flooded out. The rooftop emergency generator continued until the fuel pump on the ground floor failed.

—Patients could not get dialysis without running water.

Chapter 5

Medical Center of Louisiana: A Confident Commander Weathers a Disaster

"About 2 a.m. Tuesday morning, we received word that the levees had failed. We began to understand the gravity of the situation that faced Charity," John Jones remembered, "We were stuck there and had no idea how long we would be stranded."

As the ugly truth circulated throughout Charity Hospital, Jones took a realistic appraisal. "We had all of the supplies we needed, the staff was well-trained, they had seen hurricanes before, and we thought someone would come and evacuate the patients."

"The National Guard, the Army—we weren't sure—but we knew that someone would come to evacuate us. We knew our patients couldn't stay here forever, especially without power and air conditioning," Jones said. "But we also knew that we were there for them, and we weren't about to leave without our patients. In fact, no patient was abandoned, and our nurses stayed with them until they were evacuated. Our nurses, including me, were the last to leave," he said proudly.

✕✕✕✕✕

John Jones was the director of nursing at the Medical Center of Louisiana New Orleans, Charity and University hospitals, when Katrina struck the South Louisiana. Jones has been retired since 2009, and in 2015 he still walks with a straight military bearing of someone who is accustomed to being in command. His grey hair and pleasant expression are accented by piercing blue eyes, and he exudes a calm outlook on life. He's slimmer since he started working out on the stair trainer six days a week. "I wasn't going to wait for the doctor to tell me I needed to lose weight," he muses.

When Jones was chosen to lead the hospital as director of nursing, he brought a varied career experience that included the Vietnam War.

He humbly describes his experience as a US Navy nurse in Japan assigned to an ICU air evac system with as many as eight patients. "Sometimes I was the only RN with a few corpsmen, and sometimes the turnover was eight a day. They were transferred in and out to hospitals very quickly, and I learned that I had a much greater capacity for work than I thought was possible," he said. "It was a lesson that I would never forget. I think I grew a lot as a nurse and a person in those days."

Brief History of Second Oldest Hospital in America

—French seaman Jean Louis bequeathed a grant in 1736 to create a hospital named "The Charity Hospital for the Poor."

—First location was on Chartres and Bienville streets in the French Quarter.

—The next 100 years will see Charity Hospital move five times and finally settle in Faubourg St. Marie, now the Central Business District of New Orleans.

—In 1939 the present hospital on Tulane Avenue was completed. It was the vision of Gov. Huey Long, and at 2,680 beds was the second largest hospital in the country.

—Charity never reopened after Katrina. Charity is boarded up and lifeless on Tulane Avenue.

—As the University Medical Center was preparing to open nearby, the Bobby Jindal administration asked for ideas in June 2015 on what to do with the huge property.

Jones brought a steady, cool command to disaster planning, and management and problem-solving. When the University campus of the downtown New Orleans Charity system erupted in a blaze that destroyed the top two floors of the hospital, he was called by the evening hospital nurse administrator at two in the morning. He witnessed scores of firemen attacking a raging fire on the top floors. The first patients he found were neatly arranged on the front lawn with their nurses in attendance.

The excitable evening administrator ran up to him, babbling, wild-eyed and reported the obvious, the hospital had fire damage, and the patients were evacuated safely.

"How many casualties?" he asked.

None, she replied.

"And anyone else in danger?"

"No, everyone is evacuated and we're taking care of them now," she said.

"Good," he said, "give me a full report in the morning." Jones returned home and went back to bed.

"There was nothing to worry about," he said, "the patients were being cared for in good form despite the fire, and the firemen looked like they had it under control, so it seemed we had nothing to worry about." His calmness was remarkable in the face of a potential disaster.

As the director of nursing. John was on the Activation Team for Katrina, and he was deeply involved in preparations. "The hospitals had a good supply of food, water, disposable supplies, and other items that past experience indicated we needed. Since John lived in Florida much of his life, he was accustomed to hurricanes. "In fact, I like the wind blowing, the rain, the lightning, and I love to see the sun come out and the water drain away after it's all over. But that's all, I don't like the damage and the injuries and the power failures. I suppose I've seen so many of them in my life and so many times endured the storm, that I'm experienced in planning to take the right steps to prepare for the events, and then not worry about it."

Most of the Activation Team shared John's calmness as Katrina approached. They focused on getting ready. "Every winter the process of evaluating the previous year's experience was put into motion, and then the following spring we would have preparation meetings, drills, tell the staff to prepare to be on one team or the other, and to make plans for their families," he said. The nursing staff "was always getting ready for the storm season and the people on the Activation Team were very comfortable with their responsibilities."

Over 1000 staff members and families sheltered at Charity during Katrina. The staff focused on taking care of approximately 480 patients.

Many overcame serious personal problems to do their jobs. "I think only two nurses out of the entire Activation Team (about 500) needed counseling" he recalled. "I know many people on the staff had very difficult personal moments, but they endured them well." Almost all of the nurses retained their professional composure through the event, but the symptoms of PTSD would emerge weeks and months later.

One staff member received a call from her children who were in the attic and the water was rising, but she kept her composure and did her job. It was like that with the great majority of the nursing staff.

"Nurses are remarkable in that sense, that we have a responsibility

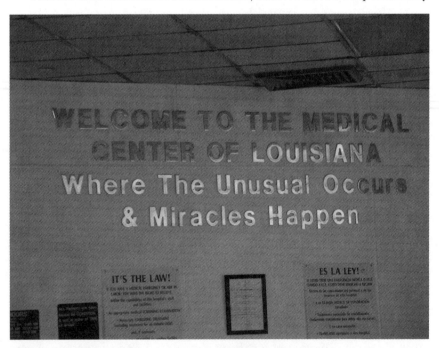

Medical Center nurses and doctors expect the unusual and sometimes deliver miracles.

to show up for work, to do our jobs, to take care of our patients, despite everything that could happen to us. We all thought it was the most important thing to take care of our patients at all costs," he said, "And that's what we did. We cared for our patients."

As Katrina approached the city that Monday morning, the rain and wind picked up very early, and the hospital experienced several hours of thunder, lightning, and torrential rain. The streets around the old hospital flooded. Later the skies cleared, the water drained away, and for a few hours it looked like it might be over.

Staff members focused on taking care of patients. On Gravier Street near the ER entrance, the infamous "smoking area" regulars speculated when they would go home.

Mother Nature and geography had played a cruel trick on Charity Hospital. Mid-City was one of the last neighborhoods to flood. As the hurricane moved north, it appeared the worst was over. And for Monday most of the media told the outside world the same.

Details of the levee failures trickled into the Office of Emergency Preparedness at City Hall, and the false hope of a quick recovery was dashed.

"As the water rose and the city flooded, including the basements in both University and Charity, it evolved into a catastrophe," Jones said, "but I don't think anyone inside the hospital knew the extent of the damage to the city. With cell towers down, it was difficult to impossible to communicate, and when power and cable went out, information was limited to reports from friends.

"I remember we found a phone in the medical building near University that for some unknown reason was working when nothing else would work. Every day a line of staff showed up and we limited our calls to about three minutes. So I called my sister in Florida and asked her to tape CNN, because we really had no way to tell what was going on," he remembered.

Although rumors were swirling around the hospital, most went to sleep on Monday night after the storm hit, suggesting they would be going home shortly. The pumps would drain the water and the Recovery Team would be coming to relieve the A Team the next day.

rose around the two hospitals that comprised the
, more sinister problems emerged. Both hospitals
trial generators, yet the rising water flooded the
ing equipment.

Charity was a Depression-era building designed with three-foot thick masonry walls built around a steel structure with many sealed windows. This design was excellent for keeping in cool air provided by air conditioning. With no power and very little effective air circulation, the massive structure started to heat up. Every operating window that could open was opened, and many windows that were considered permanent were knocked out.

The morgue and the central kitchen were both located in the basement, and as the power failed, both lost all refrigeration. The elevators stopped.

Charity lost power and city water. Some suburban hospitals, like Ochsner Medical Center had the foresight to drill artesian water wells. The state hospitals did not have wells. The life-sustaining fresh running water was now gone— for the plumbing system, for lab tests, for dialysis, for surgery, for hygiene. The pallets of bottled water that were brought into the hospital before the storm would quench the thirst of patients and staff for days, but were not suitable for many other medical needs. And with no air conditioning, the amount of water required per person would only increase.

Restrooms needed creativity. With no water to flush toilets, and the city sewerage system at a standstill, the staff used the legendary Charity talent for improvisation. They converted five-gallon buckets into toilets. Temporary restrooms were established in seldom-used rooms away from normal traffic to isolate the accompanying fragrances. Regular trips to the water closet had now morphed into an exotic adventure in urban bathroom hygiene improvisation.

Jones remained unshaken. His calm demeanor was intact. If ever an emergency required calm nerves and a cool leader, he was the leader.

"I had the unshakable belief—it was always with me—that we would be all right after this period of discomfort," he remembered.

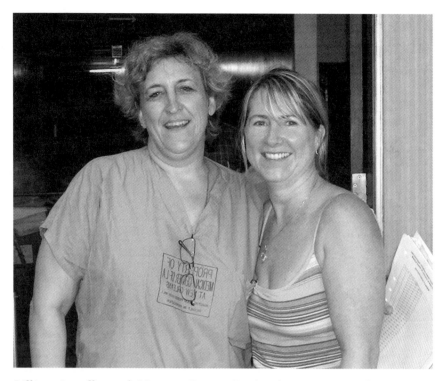

Lillian Agnelly and Mooney Bryant-Penland, nurses at Charity Hospital during Hurricane Katrina.

"I had absolute confidence that the nurses would do the right thing. Nurses are remarkable in that sense, that we have a responsibility to show up for work, to do our jobs, to take care of our patients, despite everything that could happen to us, we all thought it was our most important responsibility, to take care of our patients at all costs. And that's what we did. We cared for our patients. No nurse abandoned a patient, rather, we lived with our patients until we all evacuated. And I don't know of a nurse at Charity who would have it any other way."

New Orleans became a city spiraling out of control. Before the day was over, the fire and police departments completely collapsed with the flooding and destruction of headquarters and assets. Several fires raged out of control in the city, natural gas and sewer lines burst, causing gushers of flames and water, and gunshots rang

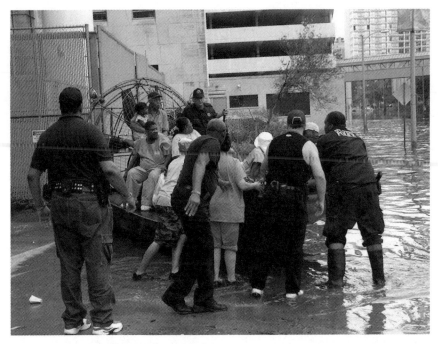

An airboat crew begins evacuating patients at Charity Hospital.

across the City That Care Forgot. Nobody knew when the water would stop flowing into the city— not the Corps of Engineers, not the city water board, and certainly not the besieged staff at Charity.

"It was hot like you cannot believe," said ER nurse John Penland, "so Monday night, my wife Mooney and I were asleep when I heard someone say, look, just like the bathtub, it's kind of swirling around. I went outside on the ambulance ramp to see a large whirlpool in the water leading into the basement wall, and then everyone came to the realization at the same time. Water was coming into the basement through the hole in the wall where the cyberbaric pipes entered the building."

They ran into the ER, and saw the water slowly working its way up the stairs from the basement. Then someone yelled out, 'The water is coming up into the ER!'"

The dauntless ER nurses had saved many a life by making interventions without a doctor's order or a textbook example.

Nobody had to tell them to evacuate their entire ER. Doctors, nurses, staff, aides—everyone grabbed medical equipment, supplies, charts, patients and ran up the stairs. The second floor auditorium had been used for training, exhibits, and meetings. Now it filled with patients.

"I've never been so hot in all my life, and God willing, I'll never be this hot again," said Lillian Agnelly, a new supervisor in Charity's ER, one of the busiest in the country. She was from New Jersey and she had had never seen the lethal combination of temperature and humidity that had Charity and her patients firmly in its grip. As everyone sweated, they had to wonder when they would leave the sweltering auditorium turned into an ER.

The nurses and staff awoke to an entirely new world on Tuesday. The rumors had turned into a horror story as radio and TV reports confirmed the worst fears of the Activation Team—the city had flooded and they were surrounded by a toxic gumbo of water, waste, chemicals, dead and decaying bodies and animals.

Tuesday had moments of promise. As the ER staff stood outside on the ambulance ramp contemplating the rising water, they were startled to see a small flotilla of the Louisiana Wildlife and Fisheries Department (LDWF) boats motoring down the street in their patrol boats. The thin-hulled aluminum *bateau* (a Cajun boat) was powered by an outboard motor. It was the standard patrol boat for wildlife officers.

The shallow-water *bateaus* were ideal for rescue. These dauntless heroes were men who had spent their lives patrolling back water bayous and rivers. Tough as gators, wily as otters, and utterly fearless. The officers saved inept boaters, trappers, hunters and lost birdwatchers. Their small boats could be launched almost anywhere that had a few inches of water. Hurricane? Yeah, so what, we've seen 'em all our lives. The Hurricane Pam exercises the year before had assigned the wildlife agency to search and rescue. Every agent was experienced and ready to do their jobs.[2]

No Category 5 hurricane would keep these agents away. They were prepared to launch within moments of the passing of the hurricane, and now motored up to the ER ramp, beached, and then asked the surprised staff: who gets out first?

The most critical patients were located in the Intensive Care Unit (ICU), and nine patients from the University Campus ICU, and four from the Charity campus ICU were considered the best candidates to send out first.

The ICU was on upper floors, but without elevators, the fragile patients would need to be secured to "spine boards" then carried down the stairs. However, there were not enough spine boards for the ICU patients. The Charity talent for creative improvisation emerged. Nurses and EMTs ripped doors from their hinges, loaded patients on the doors, and husky officers carried them down the heavy-duty steel fire escapes to the patrol boats with nurse escorts.

The sudden appearance of the wildlife officers was exhilarating. The beleaguered Charity staff hoped that help was on the way.

Their hopes were buoyed at 3 a.m. Wednesday. LSU was ordered to triage patients for evacuation, and at 11 a.m., Charity was notified their evacuation was to begin in 30 minutes. By 4 p.m. no evacuation was in sight. Later that evening, they were notified that the water was too high for the National Guard trucks.

Hope and salvation vanished, only to be replaced with doubt and fear.

On Thursday, August 31, Charity staff heard more bad news. Evacuation orders were placed on hold again. Their evacuation was paused due to "security concerns." Reports of gunfire echoed throughout the city.

"It was like the rug was pulled out from under you," John said, "one minute you are getting everyone ready to evacuate, and the next moment you are not. That hurt."

The staff had gone from euphoria at the prospect of evacuation to a kick in the stomach, and the dreadful specter of spending another night in the biggest hospital-turned-sauna in the world. "It was difficult for people because one moment you are getting ready to go out of the door and the next it was slammed shut. But I had absolute confidence that our nurses would do the right thing. I had faith that everyone would continue to do their jobs."

"In this extraordinary event, the administration knew that we had to hold everything together, and we did our best to communicate, communicate and communicate to everyone. We held meetings for all staff at 7 a.m. and 5 p.m. to update staff regardless of what there is to report, even if it was simply rumor control—and there were some fantastic rumors—the meetings were worth it. We would yell up the stairs that the meetings were about to start, and to send a representative to the meeting. It did get rather tiresome for staff that had to go up and down several flights of stairs, but the meetings were well worth it because when everyone was informed they felt more confident that action was being taken to help the hospital."

Looking back at the environment of sweltering tropical heat, a loss of modern hospital services, and an extremely challenged staff, John said he witnessed many extraordinary events. "From the upper floor of the hospital, we could see a city of total chaos, fires burning out of control, thousands of people wading, walking, swimming and floating on everything you can imagine," he said.

"I remember being on the fifth floor of University looking down at the street and saw this man paddling along on a door. He fell off, but got back on, then fell off again and went underwater, he came up once, then went under again and didn't come back." John recalled a sinking feeling, "I felt so helpless. There was no way I could get to him. Nobody to call to help him. He just disappeared under the water and never came back up."

"People just did incredible things I'll never forget. For example, the elevated interstate was only a few feet above the walkway that connected Charity to University. People were so desperate to get off the interstate; they tried to jump on to the roof of the walkway. OK, but they landed on the roof of the walkway. Many of them lost balance and then slid into the water. It was not very far down to the roof, but a good 15 feet to the water." The water was six feet and deeper.

Thousands upon thousands, perhaps 100,000 people, were up against the fight of their lives. Rising water in the city caught many unprepared. They couldn't imagine such a catastrophic flood, but what could they do?

It was the end of the month and many of the city's poor were flat broke.

Desperate families clung to anything that floated—big plastic containers, wash tubs, doors, and air mattresses. They threw the kids in it, a few meager possessions, and struck out for high ground. Some people didn't make it.

※※※※※

John worried about his own safety only once—when he was on the walkway connecting University hospital to the Seton medical office building. He had seen many helicopters in the Navy, and knew that they don't always leap into the air. He was looking at a helicopter on the roof of University trying to take off with a full load. As it slowly rose, "the craft started to turn toward me, and as I saw the vertical rotor coming around, the thought occurred to me, *What if it doesn't get up, and comes down? Then it could land on me!* So I quickly retreated from the walkway and moved into the building."

Describing the torrid heat, momentous uncertainty, and a staff that was virtually glued to their sweltering wards, John observed, "I was concerned about my nurses, but they made me proud of them. I knew most of them well enough to look for signs that they were having difficulty meeting the demands of the conditions we faced, but we all persevered. The great majority of our nurses are all heroes, there is no doubt in my mind, but they weren't the only heroes."

Patients could die with no electricity for their mechanical ventilators or other critical medical devices. The facilities and maintenance staff was prepared. They placed a number of smaller, portable generators in strategic locations around the hospital and ran extension cords to the most vital machines that absolutely had to keep running.

"We knew fuel would eventually run out, but some of our nurses reconnoitered the parking lot with what they told me was the 'Mississippi Credit Card.'

"What's that? I asked, and the proud scrounger showed me a surgical hose they used to siphon diesel fuel out of any vehicle, including ambulances, they could find parked in the garage."

※※※※※

In the birthplace of Creole cuisine, humble New Orleans residents sneered at white bread sandwiches, Kool-Aid, and other common American staples.

Here's what some Katrina staff brought to eat during Katrina: Fried chicken, daube glace, smothered pork chops, sautéed trout, crawfish étouffée, was the menu on the minds of the families and staff. Even the most basic plate of red beans was amplified with hot sausage, pork chops, boudin, grilled ribs, or smoked delicacies. If they had to spend the weekend away from home, well then, they would bring the best part of home with them.

"Activation Team members were allowed to bring family into the hospital to stay during the storm, but some were not as well behaved as the patients," John said, "Of course, this is a city that revolves around food, and everyone brought every kind of food you can imagine with them to the hospital. And they brought with them every type of cooking device to properly prepare the vittles. There was fried chicken in the admit area, ice chests everywhere, and people tried to smuggle into the hospital hot plates, barbecue pits and microwave ovens." Charity Hospital police officers were experienced in handling the chefs of the Activation Team. More than one illicit device was ruled out of order and some were confiscated.

Musing on the staff's desire to dine just like they would at home, John said, "I'm sure that more went on than I know about because you could smell food everywhere you went in the hospital. Eggs, bacon and biscuits in the morning, fried chicken all the time, but how could you blame anyone for trying to maintain normalcy in their lives simply in order to relieve the stress of the situation?"

(Less than a year later, the Joint Commission on the Accreditation of Hospitals reviewed hospital disaster plans following Hurricane Wanda. They recommended staff relatives should not be allowed into the hospital during the storm.)

The mysterious off-and-on evacuation plans, the stifling heat, the simple lack of running water all worked mischief on the minds of the marooned. Nobody could understand why they were not evacuated when the national media reported they had already been saved. The heat, the questions of evacuation, and the uncertainty took a brutal turn on Wednesday.

"We started hearing reports on the radio," John said, "that we had been evacuated, that the very hospital we were standing in was evacuated. But we knew better because we were still there and we didn't see any evacuation. That was reported several times in the media and it was a real morale buster, but the staff responded to the false reports in typical Charity style."

LSU staff made large, colorful, hand-decorated bed sheet posters telling the world that they were still there, still alive, and certainly still kicking. A good example, someone remarked, of residents with too much time on their hands.

The posters gave the world defiant, poignant messages with a twist of humor. Making a play on words of old hospital clichés was too much fun for the artists to resist.

Trauma surgery produced *Katrina Can't Tear Us Apart* and *X-ray says All Clear. Radiology Survives* wrote another.

Other poster bed sheets were more direct: *Survived the Beast*, and *God of Abraham—Lord Please HELP this city.*

The ER celebrated its epic flight to the third floor with a sheet that read *Emergency Dept. rises above*, and created a large poster voicing their determination to persevere in the difficult circumstances, *Charity Hospital & ER Dept. LSU & Tulane, 8-31-05, Continues to Serve First Ones In—Last Ones Out—Let The Games Begin. CHNO-1, KATRINA-0.*

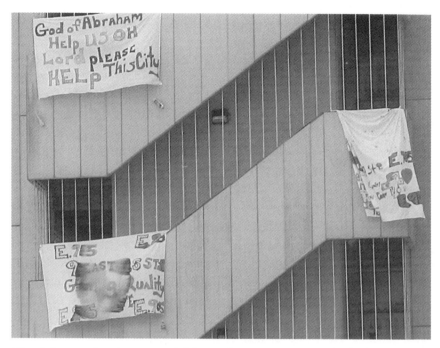

The false media reports of Charity's evacuation stoked the creative energies of marooned staff. They fashioned large bed sheets hung on the upper floors of the fire escape that could be seen blocks away.

✹✹✹✹✹

Thursday became another day with a promise of rescue—but an absence of action. "I was up early Friday morning, maybe 5 a.m., looking out toward the expressway, and saw a long line of headlights moving down the I-10 interstate toward Charity. I knew they were coming to get us," John said. Finally, he thought, we're leaving.

It was all over rather quickly, John remembered, maybe two or three hours after the trucks pulled into the ER ramp, the patients, relatives, and exhausted staff all loaded into the trucks, then moved out. A ferry system of air boats and bateaus made continuous runs from the Charity ER ramp to nearby Loyola Avenue, where everyone boarded a truck headed for the Louis Armstrong New Orleans International Airport in Kenner, west of New Orleans. At

University, a steady flow of helicopters snatched patients from the roof and ferried them to the airport.

"I was one of the last people out of the University campus," John said. "Most everyone was trucked out to the airport, exhausted, some people a bit disoriented, some of us just stunned, and for the first time in days we only had to worry about ourselves. We had been prepared and ready to move our patients at short notice for days, and now we were being put on a flight to God knows where— and most of the time nobody knew where we were going and what would happen to us. But we were out of there."

"It was kind of anti-climactic," John said, speaking of the sudden departure Charity, and then the sudden flight out of the city. "Here we were standing in the airport, exhausted, on our last reserves of energy. The airport resembled a huge triage area and MASH unit, and it hurt us to walk through all of those people who needed help. We were simply so worn out, physically, and mentally drained, that I don't how much help we could have been to them. But it hurt us just the same to see those people and not be able to help them."

His feelings of being marooned in a giant broken city hospital were soon replaced. He was now a bewildered refugee landing in San Antonio.

In the next week John would drive to Houston, Lafayette, Baton Rouge, back to Houston, and then fly to Atlanta where his brother lived. His odyssey would continue until November when power returned to his home. The memories of the storm, its aftermath, and his displacement were firmly entrenched in his mind.

He looked at the Charity crisis again with the benefit of hindsight. "That was unforgivable, the government waiting five days to get us out of Charity. One excuse was gunfire made the situation too dangerous. And the water was too deep, but in the end, it was still unforgivable."

When remembering the traumatic days of heat, uncertainty and fear, Jones said a major lesson learned has been demonstrated by a more rapid response to disasters since Katrina.

The great majority of the staff of Charity and University hospitals suffered the same experiences—and many still have the symptoms of PTSD.

The hospital itself reopened as a MASH unit in the parking lot next to University Hospital, then moved to the Ernest Morial New Orleans Convention Center, then moved to an abandoned retail store by the Superdome, and moved again to a parking lot outside of University Hospital.

The original Charity Hospital building remains closed to the public. The state of Louisiana has plans to build a new hospital in nearby Mid-City adjacent to the new VA hospital.

The empty shell of Charity Hospital is a hulking reminder of the tragedy of Katrina, but it is also a reminder of the selfless nurses and healthcare staff that suffered to care for their patients. A group of nurses who were willing to face death rather than leave a patient to die alone. A group of nurses and staff who are nominated for the title of Angels of Katrina.

Lessons Learned at Charity

—When the elevators failed, Charity nurses and staff moved patients on spine boards or by strapping patients to doors or cubicle dividers.

—Painted bedsheets hung from Charity windows with requests for help, expressions of hospital pride and even team messages.

—Charity staff prepared patients for evacuation Wednesday and Thursday. Rescues were scrubbed on both days. The water was too high for National Guard trucks. Gunfire erupted nearby.

—About 1,000 Charity staff worked and sheltered at the hospital, caring for about 480 patients. Families were allowed. A year later, the Joint Commission on the Accreditation of Hospitals recommended that family members of hospital staff should not be allowed during a disaster.

—Flotillas of wildlife agents were among the first to rescue critical patients and attending nurses in shallow-water *bateau* boats.

—Charity staff and their families brought their love of food—and cooking equipment—to the hospital for duration. Fried chicken, boudin, seafood, red beans and rice. Security allowed some cookers and boilers and turned others away.

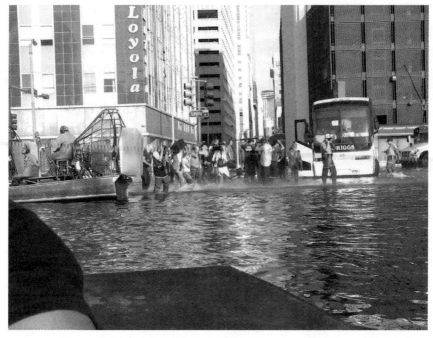

Charity nurses are evacuated by airboat to buses on Loyola Avenue.

Chapter 6
Charity Hospital Staff Pulled Together

John Jones, director of nursing at both Charity and University hospitals, had a view of events from the top down, but Cameron, an RN, had a different view of the unfolding events at the Medical Center of Louisiana in New Orleans. He was normally assigned to work on the fourth floor unit of the massive hospital known for decades simply as Charity. Cameron asked that his last name not be used in this story. The floor was only a few seconds up by elevator from the legendary ER, and served a number of functions secondary to the emergency room.

As a member of the Activation Team, Cameron went to work on Sunday morning, August 28, 2005 and worked on the emergency surgery unit. Although Mayor Ray Nagin, had called for a mandatory evacuation of the city that Sunday, Charity had been in Code Grey status, which was normal practice for an approaching hurricane for many hospitals in the Gulf South. Katrina would change many of the previous practices for disaster staffing, but for the moment, staying with old practices that worked was the game plan.

"Up until Saturday, some of it [the media] had the storm going to Florida; some of it had it going to Texas. As it got nearer to us, the projections all hit right at the mouth of the Mississippi River. So we knew it didn't look good, Cameron said. "And the size of the thing was scary! I mean, it was the size of the Gulf of Mexico with rain bands and everything. We knew we were in for a ride," he remembered ruefully.

The state's disaster activation trigger was when the hurricane was 60 miles south of the Mississippi River mouth. Hurricanes in New Orleans and South Louisiana could sometimes turn into a three-day affair that was a party attitude. Even though the hospital might be running on generators, things seemed fine with the veteran staff.

The Activation Team consisted of some administrators, some staff, but mostly nurses. This team had the duty to care for patients and essentially run the hospital until all danger had passed. Most shifts were eight hours, but during the Code Grey the shifts were divided into 12 hours to reduce the number of staff required to run the hospital. Hurricanes usually caused two or three days of service disruptions before administrators decided the conditions were safe enough to resume public service.

The Recovery Team returned after the storm to relieve the A Team. The Recovery team had no special temporary location, but its individual members stayed safe, high and dry until the storm passed. A day after the storm had passed and conditions in the hospital were deemed safe for continuing patient care, the Recovery team would be ordered return to the hospital and the A Team would go home. The A Team would then recuperate before returning to the regular schedule.

As an A Team member Cameron had already worked on Saturday. "My family, including my son, daughter-in-law and grandbaby, had gone to Texas. I caught up with them at 3 a.m. They didn't know anyone there so they had hotel reservations made. So my family and the three dogs went to Houston," he remembered.

The wind built. By Sunday evening after the sun went down, the staff would take breaks to go outside to have a smoke in the area of LaSalle and Gravier streets. The unofficial smoking area was a stone bench near the corner. The wind was blowing sand in the air, and, by seven or eight, Sunday night, the sand was hitting hard enough to be painful.

The wind would continue to accelerate Sunday evening in New Orleans until it reached category 5 of the Saffir-Simpson Wind Scale. Cat 5 is 157 mph or higher, which is the level of catastrophic damage to a city. However, the tall buildings and in the medical district of the city impeded the air flow, making it hard to determine the direction the wind.

"Then the storm hit around 7 a.m. in the morning," Cameron remembered, "It was still dark; I've heard howling like that before, so it was a really, really bad storm." Before the eyewall of hurricane reached the eastern boundaries of New Orleans, the medical district was receiving Cat 5 winds, well over 160 mph. Wind at this speed was easily capable of blowing the windows out of east side of the building and sucking the windows out of the west side of the hospital.

In conditions of very heavy wind that could shatter windows and blow debris into the patient rooms, it was necessary to take all the patients on the windward side of the hospital to the center of the hallway for safe shelter. Despite the wide halls, the unit had 20 patients lined up in the hallway, with just enough room to walk between the beds.

"One guy had a tracheotomy. All of a sudden we needed to suction him. We were running around, "We have to suction! We have to suction!' However, the power was off by then and we were on emergency generator. Charity is an old place and not everything was working. Maintenance men tried to get the emergency outlets working and so extension cords were running all over the floor. The crash cart had a portable battery-powered suctioning machine and it was charged. So we were able to suction him and he got better.

"At that point we were after the storm but before the flood on Monday. I went outside and that's when I took pictures of Charity and pictures of Tulane. It looked like there had really been a bad storm. There was a restaurant in front of Charity, and we called it the "Fistula." It had an atrium over it with glass but it was all blown clear out to Tulane Avenue. The streets were wet, and there wasn't any standing water."

※※※※※

The breech of the levees started as rumors, but then WWL-Radio and WWL-TV, New Orleans, broadcast the story that the levees on

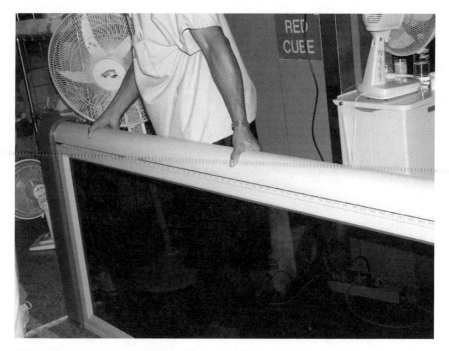

Charity nurses used office cubicle dividers as spine boards.

the 17th Street Canal and the Industrial Canal had burst. Many Charity staff members lived on the east side of the Industrial Canal so they all knew that could only mean that neighborhoods in the Ninth Ward and New Orleans East were flooding. The Activation team watched as the water encircled the hospital and rise over the sidewalk. By nightfall, the refugees streaming past Charity were chest deep in water.

Rising floodwater crippled the hospital's vital support systems one by one.

The hospital power switching equipment was located on the first floor and the basement. As power was shorted out by the rising water, heating, ventilation, air conditioning, food storage, elevators, the hospital lab, the morgue, and all the pumps went out. In a few minutes, Charity's lifesaving technology was stopped dead.

"Something as minor as the Accu-Chek machine [blood sugar test] ran on batteries. So they worked for a while, but even though they were still working, nobody had realized they've linked up to the computer. So when you put it on its cradle, it links up to the hospital's computer system, and later, you can actually go into the lab computer and find all the Accu-Cheks that have been done on the patients. Nice, except they only hold about 38 or 40 Accu-Cheks before they have to be downloaded, but they shut themselves down. But there is no way to tell if this is accurate because you can't do the test so we were cheating!"

In a city known for its wonderful food, Cameron was disappointed in the Charity menu. "Dietary, bless their souls, was feeding everybody the same thing. Whatever was the patient got, we knew that within an hour or so we would get the same thing. While the generator was still up and running [Monday], some of the nurse aides fried sausage, and we had sausage and grits for breakfast Monday morning on a hot plate." But then the power went out. So no more hot plate.

Monday was the first night without full power at Charity. The night nurse relieved Frank and he went to lie down in bed. Frank was a colleague of Cameron's. He asked that his last name not be used in this interview. The night nurses who were sleeping when the storm hit were describing the wind. They were sleeping in a bed with the head at the window, which was not a wise choice. "All of a sudden the window went out of the building. But it all went out and, thank goodness, nothing blew in," Frank said.

As the nurses became acquainted with the nursing in another century, the absence of electricity changed their practice. The Pyxis medication machine needed power to work but the Quality Team nurses said it was not a problem. "All we have to do have to do is unlock them in the back and all the drawers open, they said, but if there were narcotics inside, they didn't open. The staff was forced to return to the old days with the Quality Team bringing down medications from the pharmacy," he said.

Losing electricity made Charity dead in the water for routine services beyond lifesaving machines, elevators and illumination. Like security alarms. Like most twentieth century buildings, the outside exits had alarms that only worked when the power was on, or until the batteries died. More people could come and go from the outside exits than could be controlled. The Activation Team needed more officers because of the nature of Charity. It was a hospital that the public was accustomed to entering and leaving at will.

If nothing else seemed to work, Frank had the luxury of a phone with an outside line. "The whole length of time I was there, you could call out if you could get an open line, which was kind of nice. Nine times out of ten, whenever somebody called my ward, one of the patients would answer. It was like having an extra secretary. Some patients were too sick but not all were too sick."

One of Cameron's patients had been beaten up in a fight and had a lacerated liver. The nurses were watching for signs of distress. Without power to operate, they could do very little to help the patient. Surgery is on the 12th floor. He needed to be moved, and no machines or power were available.

The humidity abated that Monday. By Tuesday the sun shone all day, water covered 80 percent of the city. Charity was 65 years old. Windows had been painted shut for years. Soon, breaking glass echoed throughout the hospital.

※※※※※

Tuesday, Charity was no longer functioning as a hospital. *Big C* had saved the lives of thousands of patients and helped give birth to thousands more.

Suddenly Charity had no dietary services, no laboratory, and the staff could not do a complete blood count. There was no power to even run the old equipment that somebody might have had hidden away somewhere.

Since Charity is 19 stories high, there was enough water in the pipes to provide pressure on the fourth floor. But after Monday, water had flowed down and Charity was out of city water.

"We had some really sick patients. We had patients that had, due to their lifestyle, liver failure, plus the fact that their lifestyle

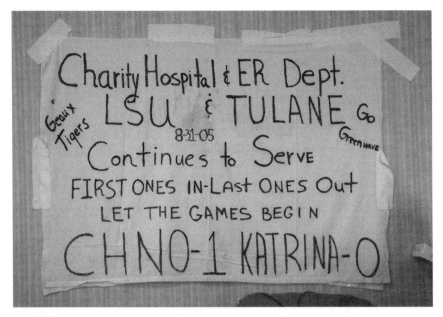

Charity Hospital nurses keep score during the darkest days after Katrina.

got them shot. So this is one guy had been shot in the arm and a leg, and the wounds had been repaired but he had an external fixate on his arm and then an incision down his leg, plus some other incisions," Cameron recalled.

"I may as well go home," he was thinking. Three times he was caught in an exit and steered back into the hospital. Apparently, the fourth time, nobody got him. "We never saw him again." The water was chest-deep outside, filled with everything in the sewers, dead bodies floating by and the patient out there somewhere with a fresh incision.

⁕⁕⁕⁕⁕

"By Wednesday, Dietary was beginning to bring us what they had in cans. Of course, they didn't have any way of heating it. So for lunch, we might get half an eight-ounce cup of cream corn and a cracker. They feed the patients first—which I understand. Then they feed us.

"They had enough nerve to come round in the morning and check and see if there are any diet changes," Frank said. "I told them, 'Everybody is supposed to get steaks now.' But no, they never did show up with the steaks. Whether they were on a soft diet, a purée diet, it didn't matter. Whatever they got, we got, and we were lucky to get it. Since we weren't able to monitor blood sugars all that well anyway, it was probably good for diabetics who were getting hardly anything to eat."

"We didn't have anything but bottled water to drink. It was just bottled water without any components at all. We called it sunlight tea...."

The portable generators were a mess. The generators had not been taken out of the crates when the storm hit. When the crates were opened and the generators set up, they didn't have any motor oil. Somebody was sent up the street to the fuel station and break-in to get oil to put into the motors. But the diesel games were not finished. Maintenance discovered that the diesel that the hospitals burned was a cruder form of diesel than the diesel generators ran and they had to go around all the parking garages and siphon diesel out of any vehicle that ran on diesel. It was maintenance and security that went out to find the diesel.

Wednesday, a group of people with guns came running up to Cameron's unit. "Everyone was saying, 'There's nothing to see here.' When you tell me that, I know that's when I'm looking at something!" Cameron said. "And after they finally cleared off, after they told us adamantly there was nothing there to see, when we opened the door and looked down, there was a body in a body bag laying down there. I don't know to this day if that was a victim of the flood, or whether it was a looter."

Bodies were found in the water around Charity.

Some bodies were stored on the outside stairwells.

Rumors flew as fast as bullets. Snipers. Looters. No cops. Men with guns.

Some of the men had M-16s and staff thought they military. One of the gunmen was dressed in street clothes. Nurses hoped he was law enforcement.

"He appeared to be because I was looking out a window, and he motioned to me that a sniper was near," Cameron said. "Whether there were really snipers, I don't know."

⁂⁂⁂⁂⁂

"As Wednesday wore on, the military appeared in Chinook helicopters with twin rotors. They would come and hover over Tulane's parking garage. We never did know what they were doing," said Cameron. "Tulane was supposed to have been evacuated by a separate entity because Tulane is a private institution. So all of its patients were evacuated by some private evacuation company. They got their own helicopters and got all the patients out."

"Then they just let the place go. They were breaking windows out. They were going all up and down Tulane Avenue, knocking out windows. There were windows out of buildings that were not out of buildings from the storm," said Cameron.

⁂⁂⁂⁂⁂

Floodwater poured into the city for four days. By Wednesday, only vehicles that could drive in water four feet or deeper were large US Army trucks. The staff kept thinking surely one of them would come to rescue them, but they just kept going by. Periodically, the big trucks would drop off water and food in small quantities, but the staff already learned to be grateful for whatever they could get. Charity was swimming in water Wednesday, but it would continue to flow into the city until it was level with Lake Pontchartrain to the north.

Thursday, Charity administrators told the staff that if the wait got any longer, they would start rationing water to three bottles of water per day per person. "With that heat three bottles was not enough. We were giving out medicine as best we could. For a patient with hypertension, nurses would dig around to take their blood pressure. We didn't have any manual blood pressure cuffs to use and all the fancy electrical stuff was dead," Cameron said, "It was like a MASH unit except MASH units would have lights and communication. We didn't have either of those."

"Communication was just improvisation at best. The location with better reception for cell phones was a roof between the third and fourth floors," said Cameron who worked on the center of the fourth floor near that roof. Since security alarms were disabled without power, it was easy to use the fire escapes and go out on the roof.

"We would go out there and stand and talk, look at the stars and cool off. It was cooler out there and I got information from a guy that ran Charity's emergency preparedness program in the emergency room," said Cameron.

Even with a source of reliable information, Frank questioned in his mind if the source was valid. Although Cameron's supervisor was going to meetings every day, he was given the same misinformation in the meetings that everyone else received. The ongoing rumor of FEMA helicopters coming to rescue Charity was a staff favorite. The story was repeated but nobody came to evacuate the staff.

"I was getting calls from as far away as my cousins out in California, saying, well, they say there's somebody coming. I said, 'I know there's no one coming because we are here!' I was getting information from people near and far. It seemed like the farther from Ground Zero you were, the more reliable information.

"From Wednesday it was like: get ready," Cameron recalled, "we're going to start transferring patients out of the hospital. So we go down there and stand around and nothing would happen. So we go back upstairs."

Friday morning the GIs arrived in actual military uniforms and airboats. Nobody had ever seen so many air boats. The airboats were circling Charity around and around.

"**The soldiers were all armed to the teeth.** They had shotguns and M-16s and apparently they were preparing to stop and start evacuating people. But they were evacuating them by airboats. Evacuating the 500 or so patients seems like an easy task, but many of the patients were not walking and the hospital did not have backboards to move patients," said Cameron.

"Usually hospitals use the backboards that are taken out of ambulances and brought into the hospital because they generally do not have a backboard for every non-ambulatory patient in the building. Nurses and staff went down to the Admitting Department and tore the interview cubicles apart to use the panels for backboards," he said.

"The last patient that left my unit weighted over 300 pounds and was paralyzed from the waist down," Cameron recalled, "and I was one of the ones hanging on to him. We took him down on a pressed wood bookshelf with four people on each side." The nurses and staff carried the patient down four flights of stairs.

"Even when the last patient had been moved out of Charity, staff had to stand in line while administrators made sure all the patients had been moved out before they could tell us that we could start leaving. Charity's footprint covers two large city blocks, so the hundreds of staff stood in a line that snaked all around ground floor, waiting to be told that we could leave," he said.

Finally word came down that all the patients were out.

"One of the protocols of moving patients, even if it's just in an airboat, the patient had to have transfer doctor's notes and, if possible, transfer doctor's orders. Due to a loss of power everything was handwritten because there were no official orders. The complete lack of power eliminated the stamping machine so that the name, ID number and complete orders were all written by hand," Cameron said.

The patients had to have all of this material with them in a plastic bag, stapled and taped to the gown before they could leave. When the patient reached the next healthcare providers, the proper information on the patient would be attached.

"When the last patient was put on the airboat, they became evacuees. When the staff was placed on a boat, they became refugees. Patients were evacuees. The staff was refugees." Cameron curiously recalled, "it seemed kind of strange that someone was adamant about making sure we were refugees.

"I don't remember eating anything Friday," Cameron said, "We were just getting the patients out. Just like rush, rush, rush! As for water, there were crates of water still sitting all over Charity." Cameron was nauseated. He thought about drinking normal saline or D5 and a half and 20 to replenish his electrolytes. He asked other nurses why they didn't drink it, and they replied they couldn't get the fluid in fast enough with running around trying to take care of patients.

"They would not let us go back upstairs. I was telling them that I needed to get my things and we finally found it already downstairs. The airboat pulls up, and they say, 'You're next.' So I put my suitcase in a boat, then some other people demanded getting in the boat first. Once again, I had to go into the boat to get my suitcase out," he said.

"The staff was standing in this huge long line in the large hallways at Charity. It was about about three in the afternoon when the line started moving, and then it took about three hours. The airboats shuttled the staff to Loyola Avenue near the US Post Office, which is several blocks away because it was dry," he said.

"FEMA told us they were taking some buses to the airport, and some of the buses were going to Baton Rouge," said Cameron. He asked which buses were going to Baton Rouge and climbed aboard that bus. Of course, it went to the airport!," Cameron said.

A police officer had to stop the bus before getting to the airport. The road was blocked by the Kenner police, and the bus driver had to get out of the bus to tell him where he was going. He got off the bus to talk to somebody, comes back and says, "Oh no, I was supposed to go to Baton Rouge." To the relief of everyone on the bus, the driver turned around in the airport entrance and headed for Baton Rouge.

"When I got to Baton Rouge, my cell phone was dead, and they dropped us off at the homeless shelter in Baton Rouge. At least the shelter had power sockets to charge my phone and call my wife," Cameron said. She purchased the last flight out of Baton Rouge to St. Louis at 4 a.m. in the next morning. Cameron almost lost his luggage at Charity, which had his camera in it because after the last patient was moved off the floor he did not know it. "I left all my things on the fourth floor. Somebody I worked with had the common decency to bring my suitcase down."

"When traveling to Baton Rouge, I checked my suitcase because it's like everybody and their dog is leaving Louisiana. Everybody is stuffed into the airplane. It was described as looking like Calcutta without the cows," he said. There was the plane and the bus was about the same. There was just enough room. Every seat was full.

"Then we left Baton Rouge and got to Houston. Once we got to Houston, things started to normal out because, like, even though there were getting all these influx of people who drove there, they weren't inundated with their own people trying to get out," Cameron said.

He arrived in the Houston airport to find his luggage didn't make it. "So they were saying they would mail it to me. But there was stuff in there I just had to have. It was all I had for a whole week and all I was likely to have for a while. And they said, the plane is supposed to be here in two hours. So I said, what's two hours after all this?"

"Nice things started happening when we got to Illinois. We're staying at my sister-in-law's house. It's a two-bedroom house and we had my wife, me, two boys, three dogs, my son, daughter-in-law and the baby. That wasn't really good in a two-bedroom house. So we went to the Baptist Church. My wife asked the lady at the church if they had a newspaper so we could look up an apartment or something to live in because we thought we would just rent an apartment, and then that would get the load off my sister-in-law.

The lady said, "Well, the parsonage is been sitting empty for about six months, and its three bedrooms."

"So we moved into the parsonage for free insisting on paying utilities and phone. We stayed there until we were able to come back down here. My son and daughter-in-law were staying with us in that house, but there wasn't a lot of space for the baby. The Red Cross ended up putting them up in a hotel They ended up staying there until we were all able to get back to Louisiana."

More strangers did more nice things, too.

"There was a pizza place we always go to when we're up there. We didn't tell anybody where we're from. In Charleston, Illinois, it's a college town, and they used to have trouble with college students drinking. Because of that, all the people in the pizza place had to be carded. We didn't say anything about where we were from, but when we got ready to leave, the lady says, 'You don't owe anything.' Another time, my daughter-in-law was shopping and then she got her nails done, just as a treat," said Cameron. "When she was finished with the nail treatment, the nails were paid for by the lady ahead of her. It was amazing how nice everyone was to us."

Chapter 7

Tulane Medical Center Acts Decisively

One of the largest hospital helicopter evacuations is credited to Hospital Corporation of America during the chaos of Katrina. Its Tulane Medical Center had nearly 1,200 patients, staff and families who needed help.

As the federal government, state and local leaders dithered, HCA and Acadian Ambulance Service company staffs mobilized.

Tulane Medical CEO Jim Montgomery ordered some parking lot light poles dismantled early in the week in case helicopters had to land. They did—soon after the evacuation was ordered the next day.

Tulane Medical's director of hospital operations George Jamison brought lessons learned from his US Coast Guard career. He gathered 1,500 pounds of cat litter before the disaster. For human toilets.

A few evacuated. More came to Tulane. As the small Acadian Ambulance helicopters carried out two patients at a time, Tulane had to accept about 70 additional patients from the nearby Superdome. They had special needs—and not much paperwork. One had a note clipped to him: "needs insulin."

Tulane's medical staff wrestled a 500-pound patient down four or five flights of hospital stairs then up to an emergency landing area atop the parking lot.

Flying a helicopter at night is hazardous enough. US Coast Guard Cmdr. Bill McMeekin landed his Jayhawk crew in an emergency landing zone with feet to spare, surrounded by tall buildings in the blacked-out city. He landed expertly with critical supplies.

✖✖✖✖✖

Medical Education Started at Tulane in 1834

The Medical College of Louisiana, the second-oldest medical school in the South, was founded in 1834, and in 1847 it became part of a newly established public institution, the University of Louisiana.

In 1884 Tulane became a private university and was renamed in honor of benefactor Paul Tulane. He was a wealthy merchant who had made his fortune in New Orleans and donated more than $1 million in land, cash and securities to the university.

In 1886 Sophie Newcomb Memorial College was established for women within Tulane University. It was named in honor of Harriet Sophie Newcomb.

The Tulane School of Hygiene and Tropical Medicine was established in 1912 and the Tulane School of Public Health and Tropical Medicine was established in 1967.[1]

Tulane Medical Center was purchased by Hospital Corporation of America in 1995. HCA was founded in 1968 by three Nashville doctors who grew the company from a small regional group of hospitals to one of the largest hospital corporations in America. HCA has correctly been credited with organizing one of the largest corporate evacuations of a hospital in history. At the time Katrina struck, the hospital sheltered over 1000 family and staff, and 178 patients.[2]

✖✖✖✖✖

Tulane Medical head of plant operations, George Jamison, a former Coast Guard Senior Chief, had a few different ideas about disaster preparations. He had 1,500 pounds of kitty litter safely stowed away for unforeseen events. He was dead serious when he said, "We have everything for an emergency around here."[3]

"What do you think we were doing with 1,500 pounds of kitty litter? Because we knew that someday we might have to use the bathroom without running water, that's why!"[4]

Jamison's experience and creativity would be hard-pressed during the hurricane. But he and his operations crew rose to the occasion again and again, earning the respect of everyone who knew them.

Danita Sullivan, Tulane chief nursing officer, was a lifelong resident of Louisiana who was worried for her staff and family. A premonition prompted her to call her sister: "OK, just in case something happens, I love you."[5]

Then she said, "I'm not scared that I won't survive. I'm scared for all of these people. We have so many people here, and I'm not sure what will happen to all of them."[6]

She sought reassurance from Jamison. She asked him if the building would stand. "He looked at me and said, yeah, it'll stand. We'll be all right." His confidence gave her the reassurance that she needed.[7]

⁂⁂⁂⁂⁂

Nathan was a veteran ER nurse who volunteered for the A Team at Tulane. He had seen hurricanes before, and was not worried about leaving his wife and children at their suburban home. He wasn't worried about this storm and thought it would be much like the others he had experienced. He asked that his last name not be used for this book.

"I work nights in the ER and was scheduled on Saturday night before the hurricane," he explained. "As I drove into New Orleans, everyone was evacuating out of the city, so I was one of the only vehicles going in. I thought how crazy I must be, but then again, I had worked through a few hurricanes earlier in the year, I forgot the names, but they were pretty much false alarms and nothing happened. I thought this would be the same."[8]

"Saturday night was pretty quiet," said Nathan, "and non-critical patients were discharged or moved into beds on the floor or CCU. The staff was instructed to move to the ER to the third floor in case of water. Most of the nurses' activities were due to the relocation of the ER. But then a sobering thought began to sink into their minds—this hurricane might be different."

"Saturday I stayed in a hotel nearby so I wouldn't need to drive home. The hospital got us a half-price rate and I slept pretty well. Sunday night was still pretty normal and not too busy since everyone was evacuated or battened down, even the ambulances weren't going out unless absolutely necessary," he remembered.

✳✳✳✳✳

"Sunday, I slept at the hospital since it was now the midst of the storm. I had a room overlooking the interstate and would check outside when I woke a couple of times. The wind and the rain were pretty intense. It blew the roof off of a bar across the street but the hospital was fine. At some point the electricity went off but the generators kicked on. When I went to work, we had emergency power and lights as well as air-conditioning, so it wasn't bad yet. We moved the ER back to the first floor and thought we had dodged a bullet again," Nathan said.

"We only had emergency power so we had no CNN or any type of news, but we began to hear about levee breaks and flooding in areas of Chalmette and the Ninth Ward. People named places and levees but I'm from California and wasn't familiar with all of the places. It was later Monday when the water began to rise outside the hospital and we had real concern." The ER was moved back to the third floor for the second time in two days.

On Monday afternoon, Tulane Medical Center CEO Jim Montgomery saw the rising water, and news reports of broken levees circling the Crescent City. He had already surveyed the top of the Tulane parking garage and noticed that only a few light poles needed to be removed to turn the garage into an emergency helicopter landing pad. "I'm not sure why I did this, to be honest, because at the time, it didn't look like we needed to evacuate, and certainly not by air. But I wanted to take a mental picture of what the place looked like," he said. "And I went up there and noticed there were four light poles that would have to come down if we were going to land an aircraft up there."[9]

HCA at a Glance

Headquarters: Nashville.

Established: 1968.

Employees: 204,000 in 2015.

CEO/Chairman 2015: Milton Johnson.

Ownership: Publicly traded as HCA; employee stock ownership programs.

Size: 165 hospitals, 113 free-standing surgery centers in 20 states and Great Britain.

HCA in Louisiana: New Orleans, Metairie, Covington, Lafayette, Alexandria.

※※※※※

Mel Lagarde was the head of HCA's Delta Hospital Division, and was the senior manager at Tulane during Hurricane Katrina. Early Tuesday morning when the magnitude of the flooding became apparent, Lagarde and Montgomery decided to evacuate the hospital.[10]

Montgomery called Acadian Ambulance Service Inc., a huge Lafayette, Louisiana emergency response company that operated evacuation helicopters, planes and fleets of ambulances. Lagarde told HCA leaders in no uncertain terms that evacuation of the patients was necessary.[11]

Without dependable news sources, the executives decided it was in the best interests of their patients to start evacuating. Both Lagarde and Montgomery were keenly aware that Tulane's status as a private hospital meant they could not depend upon the government to rescue them. HCA would be required to pay for a very expensive air evacuation.

HCA CEO Jack Bovendor agreed with the assessment of Lagarde and Montgomery. "We knew there was a chance the cavalry would show up, but we decided on Tuesday morning. We were going to take responsibility for this ourselves and assume the worst. We were going to assume that no one was going to come to our rescue."[12] Montgomery called Acadian Ambulance Service.

Acadian Air Med Services coordinator Mike Sonnier reacted instantly, "I already had helicopters on the way to New Orleans, and I diverted a couple of them to the hospital. We didn't have much time to think about this, so we just did it."[13]

Sonnier dispatched BO-105 helicopters that are configured for advance life support for two patients, a medic and a pilot. This limited load would mean a slow evacuation, but for the moment it was a huge ray of hope for the over 200 patients and over 1000 family and staff.

The private helicopter evacuation started Tuesday afternoon with three Acadian helicopters. Although the BO-105 helicopters were extremely limited in the number of patients they could carry, it was clear that progress was being made in moving the most critical patients to safety. Tuesday all of the babies, the children, and critical care patients were evacuated to HCA hospitals in Lafayette.

About Acadian Ambulance Service

—**During Hurricane Katrina**, Acadian Ambulance Service flew the first private medical evacuation helicopters from New Orleans hospitals.

—**Acadian Ambulance Service was founded in 1971** in Lafayette in the midst of a nationwide crisis due to new federal regulations that prohibited funeral home hearses from emergency transport.

—**The company started with three young co-founders**, two ambulances and eight medics covering Lafayette Parish.

—**By mid-2015, Acadian had over 4,000 employees** and a fleet of more than 400 ground ambulances.

—**CEO 2015:** Richard E. Zuschlag.

—**Acadian owners** established an employee stock ownership plan in 1993.

—**Acadian trained the first Emergency Medical Technicians** (EMTs) in Louisiana, and benefited from the experience of medics returning from the Vietnam War.

—**Acadian expanded Air Med Services** in 1981 to quickly reach emergency situations onshore and offshore.

—**Acadian Air Med was the first Gulf of Mexico** service with helicopters equipped with some equipment found in emergency rooms and flight paramedics. Acadian began providing contract medics for offshore energy platforms.

—**Acadian has six divisions specializing** in emergency care, air evac services, air transportation, executive charter, home and business security and EMS training.

—**The Acadian fleet in 2015** consisted of six helicopters, and three fixed wing aircraft that are configured to carry patients across the state or the nation. Acadian's Executive Aircraft Charter Service uses some of the same aircraft for business or pleasure charters.

—**Acadian has grown by internal expansion** and acquisition of other emergency services in Louisiana, Texas and elsewhere.

Source: Acadian Ambulance Service 2015.

❋❋❋❋❋

Later Tuesday morning the generators stopped. Tulane turned dark. Like many other generators in businesses and homes in the

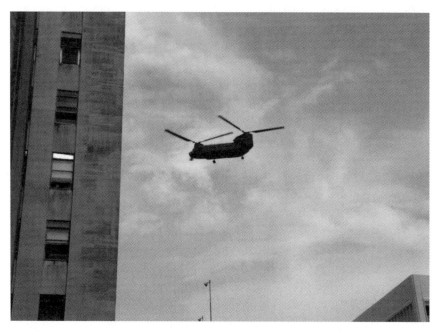

Helicopters are a welcome sight for hundreds awaiting rescue from Charity and University hospitals.

city, they had been placed on the first floor and were flooded by rising water.

Tulane Medical Center then received notice that approximately 70 noncritical special-needs patients were being transferred to Tulane from the Superdome. These patients and their families were put in the lab where space was available.

"Most came with very little paperwork," Nathan explained. "Some patients had as little paperwork as a note pinned on them saying "needs insulin." Tulane staff decided not to officially admit them—just to take care of them. Fortunately, most were patients with chronic diseases that they and their families had dealt with for years."

Nathan looked back at how healthcare staff adapted quickly in the disaster. "The pharmacy was awesome. I told the pharmacist that I needed insulin for a patient and he just handed it to me without an order or anything. I then handed it to the patient. They assured me they had syringes and everything else that they needed and we let them self-care. Some nurses, especially the least experienced, were a little uncomfortable with it at times."

Katrina had transformed the entire level of care into a mode of disaster survival. Precious little power to operate sophisticated medical equipment, water supply suddenly dry, bacteria everywhere. The level of clinical experience of the nurses became the operative factor guiding care. "My nurse manager had already given myself and one other RN access to the Pyxis machine," he said. "Access was gone when the electricity went off so she showed us how to access the non-controlled meds. She knew we could be trusted."

"One of the residents was sent up to assist us. He and I had worked previously. He handed me several vials of morphine and told me to keep the patients comfortable. We had some post-op patients, other patients with different kinds of pain. We assessed their pain on the pain scale and then gave them appropriate amounts starting with 2 mg followed with another 2 mg if they were still in pain. I was accustomed to giving boluses [doses] of 10 mg but we didn't know these patients so we used a lot of judgment," Nathan said.

The nurses were ripped from 21st century nursing care and thrust into primitive conditions as bad as a battlefield. Few of them had ever experienced a crisis like this one. "Again some nurses were uncomfortable but I told them to trust their judgment. They know what they're doing—the doctors wouldn't have given us the latitude if it weren't warranted. In a way it was nursing practice at its best," he said proudly, "We were doing what nurses know how to do and doing it well."

"The [medical] helicopters were all privately arranged by the hospital—no federal help at all. The good part was that as the helicopters came in, they brought supplies so we never wanted for anything. We had plenty of food and water. We had medical supplies brought in as well."

The physical nature of the patient was not the only factor involved in moving patients to the helipad. "Transporting patients was difficult. A respiratory therapist would hand-bag the patient, some of which were loaded in an employee's pickup truck for the journey to the roof. Good progress was made with evacuations on Wednesday but then they had to be shut down. These medical helicopters weren't equipped for night flying and there was shooting."

The evacuations continued as medical helicopters landed on the hospital parking garage. "On Wednesday, we were told that we would evacuate the hospital, and started bringing the patients downstairs so they could be taken to the parking garage via the walkway over the street," said Nathan. Not all of the patients were easily moved to the parking lot landing pad. "We had a 500-pound post-op gastric bypass patient that had to be carried down 4 to 5 flights of stairs in the hospital, then across the garage and up the ramp to the helicopters landing on the roof." Then someone figured out that the patients could be loaded in the back of a pickup truck and driven to the rooftop landing site.

On Wednesday, Charity Hospital doctors brought four critical patients to Tulane, and the patients were evacuated by helicopter. **The next day, Tulane staff helped Charity** evacuate more. On Thursday, Charity Hospital doctors asked Tulane if they could help evacuate 20 more critical patients. Mel Legarde said yes, just bring them over in small groups. That afternoon, Charity doctors and nurses arrived at the Tulane garage with about 40 patients. The helicopters configured for medical use were being directed to other hospitals at that time because Tulane had evacuated its patients. The patients were forced to wait until a medically-configured helicopter arrived.

By Thursday afternoon the medical helicopters that could carry a stretcher had been replaced by large military helicopters that were configured for ambulatory patients. These helicopters were only authorized to fly 15 miles away to the Louis Armstrong New Orleans International Airport—where conditions were much worse. Like the Superdome, the airport was an accessible drop point for military helicopters, so thousands of evacuees gathered there. Some left well-staffed but besieged hospitals for a chaotic human depot. The airport reopened to humanitarian flights August 30.

Tulane did not have control over the military helicopters from the National Guard or Coast Guard. It was not until 9 p.m. before the Charity patients were evacuated.

Dr. Bennett P. DeBoisblanc was furious. "It was hard for me to watch helicopters taking off and landing for the ambulatory patients while we had critical ill patients there. I have since heard the explanation for this, and I understand it, and it makes some sense. But as far as why I got testy, you have to understand that these patients were my moral and ethical responsibility, and I took the Hippocratic Oath to defend the interests of these people. So I thought the right thing to do was to see that the squeaky wheel got the grease."[12]

"Later, Lagarde said, "he was mad at me and I was mad as hell back at him. We definitely traded words to say the least." At that time there were about 1000 patients and staff at the Tulane garage Thursday afternoon. "By this time I had no shortage of people bitching about not being able to get on helicopters," Legarde said.[13]

After the critical patients and regular ambulatory patients were evacuated, the cavalry arrived in the form of four Coast Guard heroes: Cmdr. Bill McMeekin, co-pilot Lt. JG. Catherine Gross, aircrew survival technician third class Bret Vogel, and AMT Randall Ripley. They flew a Coast Guard HH-60 Jayhawk helicopter in New Orleans at night.

Paramedics asked McMeekin to deliver about 1000 pounds of emergency medical gear to Tulane, even though it was not clear that the medical center had a landing site. The paramedics directed McMeekin down the streets of the medical district in New Orleans. The Tulane landing site was surrounded by 200 foot, high-rise buildings closely on three sides of its parking garage. On the fourth side, but across the street from the garage, was another high-rise office building. The Jayhawk's 54-foot diameter rotor blades and 65-foot length made for a narrow squeeze between office buildings on all sides of the emergency parking lot-landing site.

Cmdr. McMeekin positioned his flight mechanic and rescue swimmer on either side of the craft as lookouts. He flew the big helicopter down New Orleans streets until he was close to the landing site. With absolutely no room for error, he piloted the Jayhawk into a "sliding, 180-degree pedal turn to a steep approach, no hover landing"—the very essence of a white-knuckle flying at night.

Cmdr. McMeekin's heroic flying was far from over for the night. The notorious hot and humid southern summer created poor flying conditions for helicopters. The big Jayhawk would be required to spring off the deck in a high-power vertical takeoff to avoid the buildings on three sides of the parking garage. The big helio leaped off the deck, as McMeekin expertly piloted the aircraft and crew to the next mission.

"The hospital security guards were real heroes," said Nathan. "They had guns and flak jackets and kept everyone safe. Patients were also brought from Charity in boats to be evacuated. There were stories of critical Charity patients waiting to be evacuated behind our employees. Not true, didn't happen. At times a small two-seater helicopter might take employees if critical patients would not fit. Most of the time the helicopter brought its own nursing staff so it could get tight quickly."

"Then they got some of the big Chinooks [helicopters] and could take several patients at once. Employees went out after patients for the most part with those with pets going last. Everyone was to be out by Thursday afternoon—but after the delay because of the shooting I knew we wouldn't make it," Nathan recalled.

The Chinook is a two-engine heavy-lift helicopter the military uses to move troops, artillery and equipment. The mission turned to saving lives.

It took until Friday a.m. to get everybody out. "By then I hadn't talked to my wife since Sunday and was beside myself with worry about her and my two children. It was a couple of very rough days worrying about them. The plan had been for them to evacuate but Sunday I learned that they had stayed in Pearl River with their family. I was really worried about them and kept trying to reach other family members who might have some word," Nathan remembered.

"On Friday, I was taken first to the New Orleans Airport and then by car to another city where we spent the first night in a shelter. At least we had a hot meal and a shower. My nurse manager found us the next day and took us to a house she was staying at. She went around and found as many of us as she could. I found out my family had gone farther north to another state and was trying my best to find a way there. I decided to check the Lafayette Airport one more time and met with the chief nurse executive there. She had just chartered a jet for a group of employees and I was able to get on. Talk about fate!" he reminisced.

"One of the happiest days in my life was when I saw my family again," Nathan said. Despite his fear for the safety of his family, Nathan said, "I would do it again in spite of that." "We were doing what nurses do, caring for patients and in a way, it was nursing at its best. We had great support from administration. I will always be loyal to this hospital. We continued to be paid and most continue to work. Although some doubt it, I think the hospital will reward our loyalty as well."

Chapter 8

Ochsner Medical Center: Well Prepared and Undefeated

The challenge of a lifetime was making a beeline for New Orleans. Ochsner was the best prepared hospital in Louisiana for a disaster. But would it make any difference to this monster from the gulf? After Hurricane Katrina thoroughly devastated the city and moved on, the ordeal was just beginning for staff.

It seemed like patients from another world. One delivered her baby in a hotel and arrived at Ochsner by boat. Another soon-to-be young mother was forced to wade through the toxic soup before finally arriving at Ochsner. A number of mothers were healthy enough to go home, but had no home to greet them. Another group of mothers were too nervous to stay at home and came to the maternity ward for safety. It was surreal.

The sterile, safe medical environment changed into a scene from a bad movie. The air conditioning failed, the elevators stopped and critical lab equipment fogged up and died. The Louisiana National Guard was patrolling the hospital just in case the urban chaos spilled over from New Orleans to Jefferson.

The total impact of Hurricane Katrina on the nursing staff is hard to measure. After working nine days in the August heat and humidity, Jackie Lupo, one of the best and brightest nurse leaders, said, "It was amazing because it seemed like a science fiction movie when you went outside of the hospital, there was no life. There was no traffic."

By any standard, Jackie had led her nurses through the worst of times. "There seemed to be no dogs, no birds on the highway outside of the city. Even though we had directions, for some reason, it was very hard to stay focused on directions. And at one point, I ended up like 30 miles away from where I should've been," she said.

It was time for a vacation.

※※※※※

Levees held around the Ochsner campus. The hospital had about a foot of water but nothing impassable.

Air conditioning failed. Every patient room was equipped with an emergency fan.

Elevators failed. Staff formed human chains to pass food up stairwells as high as the 11th floor.

When food grew short at well-stocked Ochsner, staff re-supplied at a nearby Walmart.

Armed National Guardsmen patrolled the campus. When the TV news about looting in New Orleans overwhelmed the maternity nursing staff, they voted. They turned off the TV.

"People die every day in hospitals, but no patient died in that period of time, which is pretty amazing," said Jackie Lupo.

Ochsner Health System is Louisiana's largest not-for-profit in 2015 that spans Louisiana and now Mississippi with 2,500 doctors, 16,000 employees, and 19 hospitals that it owns, manages or partners with others.

This is the story of how the Ochsner maternity ward at the main campus struggled with Katrina.

Everyone survived.

※※※※※

Ochsner Medical Center is generally regarded as one of the best hospitals in America. It is also one of the best-prepared hospitals for hurricanes. Jackie was a senior administrator at the hospital. This is her story about why things worked, didn't work and lessons learned. Her story provides insight into experiences of the nursing staff in a disaster.

During Katrina Jackie Lupo was the administrator of the maternity unit where mothers come to deliver their babies. She is a petite nurse with a bubbly personality who interacts pleasantly with patients, staff and executives. Jackie is highly-regarded at Ochsner, a member of the executive team and serves as house supervisor.

On Friday afternoon, August 26 as Katrina approached, Jackie and other managers and directors made sure the A Team and the B Team members knew what their responsibilities would be. All employees could call for a recorded update on the current hospital situation and their responsibilities. Team members would plan to stay at the hospital until all threats were past.

"Employees that are deemed essential personnel had an opportunity to choose. They could be on the A Team, the team that would come in before the crisis and stay for the duration, or they could opt for the B Team, the recovery team that comes in when the crisis is over," she said.

Saturday, Jackie was already at work at 6 a.m. She was house supervisor that day meaning her job extended beyond the normal unit to most of the hospital nursing staff. The first person said to her, "Well, what are you going to be doing during the storm?"

"And my answer was, 'What storm?'"

"Because on Thursday and Friday, it didn't look like it was much of a threat to worry about. And I had had a particularly busy Friday afternoon and evening. So I had not listened to a radio or TV after I left work that day," she said.

When Jackie arrived there was a sense of anxiety building up in the hospital. By 11:30 a.m., there were so many phone calls that Jackie asked for somebody to come in and help her staff the phones. She could no longer make routine rounds with patients in the building to see what their needs were because everything was focused on just what was going to happen the next day.

All A Team members must arrive for 7 a.m. the next morning and be prepared to stay several days, the recording said. "And we automatically went to the mode of the A Team is in and everybody else is out," she said. "The A Team was on duty and Saturday the managers were in."

The rest of the staff came in Sunday morning at 7 a.m. The day started out with meetings including some of the night shift people. Many of the night staff were already in the building and were waiting to see what would happen. The rest of the staff came in with their suitcases and their pets and their families, although pets were discouraged. But as most other local hospitals learned, Jackie said, "if that was the only way that somebody could come to work, then the hospital allowed families and pets."

The hospital discouraged the presence of families, and Jackie understood why. "You want your family as far away as they can be because that is one less thing you have to worry about. I totally understand the reasoning now. I had no family with me as my kids are older, and so it was easy for them to be away."

Jackie empathizes with the young nurses who had small children. In particular, she had one nurse who lived in the area, a nursing mother, and she chose to be on the A-Team. She stayed with her team and fortunately, was close enough that she could go home. "I just said to her 'You have to leave. There's no way you can stay here with your baby.'"

"I went home Saturday evening and actually packed a suitcase like I had done many times in the past with three sets of scrubs and some shorts and a pair of pajamas, not ever thinking that I would not be back home by Tuesday or Wednesday at the latest," she mused. "Sunday was beautiful outside. It was hard to really imagine that a hurricane was really going to be that much of a threat."

⨯⨯⨯⨯⨯

As Katrina approached, Ochsner managers met every few hours so that everyone would be informed. A schedule was needed for the 18 nurses who were on the unit to determine who would work the day shift and who would work nights. The shifts were 12 hours from 7 a.m. to 7 p.m. and the nurses chose how they wanted to work. Those who wanted to be on days started working and the night shift was allowed to relax.

"Everybody got territorial about where they would place their things and who would sleep where. A nurse on the day shift would match the night shift person for the mattress so that somebody was always occupying the space. Some of the nurses slept in the lounge and some of them slept over in the clinic, which is adjacent to our facility and was not being used at the time," she said.

Saturday evening, patients were watching TV and some could be discharged who wanted to go home. And on Sunday, a few told Jackie they didn't want to go.

"But we had a few patients there, and some of them had no place to go with their new babies. Even though they were no longer requiring nursing care or medical care, they had no place to go, so we just continued to take care of them as though they were patients. At one point for some of them, staff disregarded the charting and vital signs every so many hours. If they needed pain medication, we would certainly provide that. If they did not need much care, staff made them a category one patient meaning they really didn't qualify to stay in the hospital, but they were not dischargeable," she said.

As Katrina smashed the Louisiana coast, Ochsner Medical Center was still more than half full with an estimated 200 patients. Jackie reported families rushed some people to the emergency room and wanted them to be admitted. Some patients were coming into the hospital who were listed as bed-rest or home-visit patients and some were on home ventilation and needed a lot of care.

"Sunday evening is when the weather really turned bad," said Jackie. "It started raining and things on the TV became a lot more intense. At some point, probably either late Sunday night or early Monday morning when the hurricane really came through it was really loud and you could hear the rain."

On Jackie's unit, outside windows gave a hint of the heavy rain. "The light was just beginning to come up," she remembered, "but it never did get sunny, and there was just a bit of light. And it was really eerie because you could see the rain and the wind and how the trees were just bending backward."

Nurses on the maternity units didn't move many patients, but there was some moving on the upper floors because the wind intensified. Patients were moved into the corridors because windows were broken by the wind. The babies were moved from the 10th floor down to the second floor because of the heat and some of the wind. Later, Jackie learned that apparently the third to the sixth floor is the safest in the hospital, and anything above that is probably more at risk for wind damage.

As Monday dawned and Hurricane Katrina rapidly moved north, the skies began to clear as the day progressed. Ochsner went to emergency power. The Jefferson Parish center is located across River Road from the Mississippi River levee. It's one of the highest parts of the New Orleans region, maybe 7 feet above sea level. Stories about flooding drifted in, and water across Jefferson Highway was rising. Rumors of looting and gunfire circulated throughout the hospital.

"In a way, I'm kind of glad that I didn't know," said Jackie. Some of the nurses were getting phone calls, but many of the others couldn't get in touch with their families because the cell towers went down. **"It was very scary that you knew that your family** was in Baton Rouge or Houston," said Jackie, "but there was no connection. They couldn't get in touch with us. We had land lines, but we couldn't reach their cell phones if they were local numbers."

Another real difficulty: some of the elevators were not on emergency power. "I remembered having to get meal trays up to the 11th floor," she said. "All the employees just got in the hall and the stairwells and passed the trays up. It was amazing, the survival techniques that can kick in and help you to think of something and be creative, very creative, when needed."

Ochsner nurses might have been territorial about where they slept. Yet the hospital staff had a spirit of cooperation among departments. Jackie recalled there was no sense of departmental divisions during the crisis. "It wasn't nursing or environmental services or pharmacy or dietary. It was just everyone, doing whatever needed to be done." Staff tried to conserve the linen, because there were not very many laundry people working. At the end of the day, we would clean the bathrooms ourselves, the ones that had been used. There was no expectation that anyone was going to come behind and take care of us. This was truly a crisis and everybody had to become part of a bigger team," Jackie said.

Ochsner Medical Center history on Jefferson Highway

—Dr. Alton Ochsner, and four colleagues, Dr. Edgar Burns, Dr. Guy Caldwell, Dr. Francis E. "Duke" LeJeune, and Dr. Curtis Tyrone, founded Ochsner Hospital in 1942 on Jefferson Highway. Their goal was to provide New Orleans residents with the highest quality healthcare.

—Dr. Alton Ochsner is one of the first researchers to identify the connection between tobacco and lung cancer.

—*US News & World Report* recognizes Ochsner as "Best Hospital" in nine specialty categories—the only Louisiana hospital to be honored.

—The Jefferson campus is a 473-bed acute care hospital.

—Over 600 doctors are employed in medical specialties.

—The Ochsner Healthcare System in 2015 has grown to 19 owned hospitals, more than 50 health centers, 16,000 employees and more than 2,500 physicians in over 90 medical specialties.

※※※※※

One of the reasons that Ochsner Medical Center was so well prepared was its previous experience working with a hospital in Pensacola that was hit by a hurricane. After that hospital did a critique of their experience with a hurricane, they shared with Ochsner what was most important to maintain a working hospital. "The administration decided we'd better make sure that all those things that were learned were followed. The hospital purchased a large amount of hurricane supplies like batteries, fans, water, and other things that could be used in a disaster," she said.

"In preparation, we stored a lot of water, lots of fuel, and each patient had their own fan throughout the entire building. There were electric fans that were given to each room by our facility. You could plug it in and it worked. It was an emergency thing in every room. There was no air conditioning, but everybody had a fan," she said.

With the heat and the exhaustion and the dehydration, water was needed more often, but it was consumed sparingly. That was an extremely difficult task because the stairwells were so hot. The staff was not being denied water, but encouraged to drink what was absolutely necessary.

"Sleeping was very difficult. Everybody was working 12 hour shifts," she said. Jackie remembered wanting to make sure that everybody was here for each of their shifts and then trying to sleep. "Maybe being 10 p.m., 11 p.m. to midnight, I'd still be tossing and turning because I wasn't sleeping in a very comfortable space. It was a patient bed or an air mattress that was very different. My mind was just on so many other things. It was so hot. It was the end of August and in New Orleans, that is a very hot time of the year," Jackie said.

Jackie's unit enjoyed a washer and dryer. Since the dryer always took longer than the washer and used a lot of power, her staff would take the clothes out while still damp. Without air conditioning, the operating rooms were so hot the staff put up a clothesline. Those nurses who only came prepared to stay for two or three days soon found out a washer was available. On the night shift when the staff was busy, they would wash clothes for the folks in the rest of the hospital. One night they hit a record of 19 batches of clothes for one night. The hospital had water for washing because it had a well. Although the water was not potable, it could be used to flush toilets, take showers and keep the washing machines going.

"Pharmacy was a bit of an issue," said Jackie. "I remembered trying to get the drugs up from the pharmacy, which was on the second floor. I don't want to say that the pixie machines were unlocked. All of the rules about waiting for verification and overrides were null and void." Whatever they needed they were able to have. Nurses still needed to logon, but staff could pretty much have access to whatever they needed. You didn't need to wait for verification like now from the pharmacy to take drugs out.

Nurses working primarily in one unit were often unaware of events elsewhere in the sprawling hospital. For instance, Jackie and her colleagues did not know that the lab could not process some of the lab results. The heat in the building was so intense that the lab equipment could not work because it had to be a certain temperature. One day in the maternity unit, the ultrasound machine was totally fogged up because of the heat. Some of the equipment that staff used every day as part of the standards of care was not available anymore.

"Most of the patients were afraid," said Jackie. A couple of patients wanted to leave the hospital, but couldn't do so. "We had some patients who said, 'Discharge me. I have a family member who will come get me and I have a place in Baton Rouge.'" Jackie remembered that "some folks were hearing what was going on in the city and how some of the other local hospitals were flooded and had no electricity. They started to get really frightened. I don't want to say they were panicky, but they wanted to make sure that we were not going to flood. There were no guarantees. We were fortunate and later found out that our facility is actually seven feet above sea level. And, by the grace of God, our levees did not breach. We maybe had a foot or so water from the hospital, but nothing that was impassable."

"The hospital had moved our generators up to the fifth floor when they renovated and built the new critical care tower. Otherwise we may have been in the same situation as some of the area hospitals that were older buildings and still had their generators on either the first floor or for some, even in the basement," she said.

"So we had water, but we were trying to conserve it. At that point, no one knew what was really going to happen," she said. Eventually, Jackie had to take off her uniform shoes off and couldn't even put them back on. She had to go to just wearing flip-flops. That lasted for several days. "For a while I tried to stay in normal hospital uniform and look like a nurse," she said, "Then I just gave up. There was no hope of being in uniform. By Tuesday we weren't hearing anything about when we would be able to leave."

"The maternity unit was getting calls from patients from all over the country. Some of the patients had been patients of Ochsner and were frightened. Some of them were near delivery. They were calling to get their records sent to them, or they wanted to establish care or have whatever they need to go see another physician," Jackie said. "It required two and three nurses manning the phones just to take care of the incoming calls."

On Tuesday or Wednesday, several needy young women came to the maternity unit. One had delivered at a hotel and was brought from the hotel by boat somewhere, and then they bought her in. Several young women living in an area that was really flooded also came in.

"One lady was very tall," Jackie said, "about 5 feet, 11 inches, and she described wading in water up to her chest. When she got there, she was exhausted. Her clothes smelled so bad all we could do was strip her clothes off and allow her to take a shower. These people were just so grateful for a clean bed," she said.

"We had several women in labor. We did an emergency C-section on a patient who lived in Kenner and could not get to her own facility," said Jackie. "Ochsner had the physicians available. There is a requirement that there be enough doctors in each specialty that should anything catastrophic happen, we can at least take care of those patients."

Medical residents helped relieve the hospital staff. Residents were in labor and delivery, gynecology, and oncology. "I thought it was very interesting that they were so helpful," said Jackie. "One physician impressed the staff. He went to the floor where his patients were. He helped with vital signs. Anything that needed to be done for the patient, it was no longer up to the nurse or the physician," said Jackie, "It was the caretaker. He made rounds, talked to all of the patients, greeted them and told them not to be afraid. He stressed that there were physicians in the house. On Wednesday or so when a lot of the employees in the hospital had run out of their medication or were sleeping or whatever was going on, he went down to the outpatient pharmacy and became a pharmacist. We said he had done every scope [of practice] that was within his realm. He provided care to patients, and then he actually went down and helped as a pharmacist. The barriers, and the boundaries and roadblocks just seemed to be gone," she remembered.

※※※※※

On Wednesday, two days after the hurricane, food became a concern. Fortunately, Ochsner is located only a few blocks from a Walmart and right across the street from a food storage warehouse. "The hospital administration contacted both companies, who said that hospital personnel can go in and get whatever we needed, because if we didn't, the Walmart and the storage facility would probably be looted," she said.

"It seemed like another miracle," said Jackie. "Here we are across the street from a distribution center for food. The hospital staff went to the Walmart and they kept track of everything that they were taking. We did have abbreviated meals," Jackie said. "One time, it was tomato soup and a piece of fruit or it was cold cereal and milk. However, at no time did anyone skip a meal or go hungry."

Those meals were offered not only to the employees but also to any family members as well as patients because a lot of the family members hadn't had time to prepare food. "Everyone was given armbands so that we could identify who they were. Staff had to wear their IDs, but all the family members of either the employee or the patient had to be arm banded so that we would know at all times who was in the building," she said.

Ochsner staff made sure that pets were also cared for. They were on the fourth and fifth floors of the parking garage. "All of the pet owners were encouraged to go and make sure their pets were watered and fed and walked appropriately," said Jackie. When the staff went to gather food, they picked up pet food. "There were rabbits and cats and dogs and birds, and whatever kind of pets that one has these days. They looked like Noah's Ark. The smell wasn't so good either, but the pets were okay."

Ochsner suppliers were doing whatever they could to deliver food, water, clothes, and toothbrushes or any of the essential items. According to Jackie, the loading dock people worked 20 hours or more a day.

Some National Guard troops were in the building, but they were to assist with security because some of the hospitals were reporting looting and other crimes. "That was an eerie thing," Jackie remembered, "because only on TV did you see that kind of activity. You could be walking down the hallway, and here would come three to six will fully-dressed Guardsmen with all of their attire, including guns and whatever else it is they carry." It was pretty frightening to think that was needed in the hospital environment inside the United States.

Although communications throughout the disaster area were often nonexistent, the communications from Ochsner managers were frequent throughout the multi-building campus. "The hospital administration met with the leadership, and then leaders would meet with the middle managers. Vital information was given to the staff so that everybody could be updated and kept in touch. It was still very difficult to reach family members who were outside of the hospital. However, the hospital computer systems never went down, so some people discovered they could email their families. When the staff realized email would work, they started communicating with their families through email. That made people feel better."

Jackie remembered that at one point the unit voted to turn the TV off because the news was all about the looting and all the negativity. "Although we were assured that we were pretty safe, the TV went off. The staff didn't want to watch it anymore."

※※※※※

Ochsner was better prepared, and its staff suffered far less than other hospitals. Still, the days just seemed to drag on. "At some point, you just lost track of time," Jackie said, "you get a little crazy." They were able to go outside to get some fresh air, but could not go too far because there were still people who were trying to come into the hospital that didn't have family or any reason other than they just wanted to be there, where it was safe, and where there was food. At some point, they ultimately had to limit who came in and who went out of the building.

"Compared to some of the other hospitals, we had things pretty good, but the relief team didn't come in until day nine." complained Jackie. "We didn't evacuate all of our patients but we did send out some of our ICU patients, and almost all of our neonatal patients. That happened on day three to four, and it was pretty quick and well-organized. A lot of the nurses from the Ambulatory Care Center helped because they were in-house, and a lot of the surgery nurses because they had teams also. Anyone who was available helped out, whether it was physicians or residents or hospital administration. They took the patients down to the first floor to the staging area. Then the helicopters started coming in and taking the patients out," she said.

"Patients who were discharged and well enough were transported via bus with staff members to Baton Rouge where they could go to the Pete Maravich Center. Then they would be triaged for the most appropriate facility after that. We had some employees who had evacuated to Baton Rouge from the B Team, and they knew everything that was going on. So they went to the Pete Maravich Center, like a lot of other volunteers, and helped with vital signs and assisting with physicals. They assisted in making sure the patients were matched up with what was available in terms of resources.

"We had an affiliation with another hospital in Baton Rouge," said Jackie. "So we started transporting our patients to those areas, and then our nurses would go over there with our patients. Some of the facilities were used to the acuity of our patients. Some of those patients had been sent to Ochsner originally from there and now we were sending those same patients back. So a lot of the nurses went and worked at those hospitals," she said.

"In our area, there were several patients that were pregnant," said Jackie. "We talked with the patients, and they did not want to be transported. They wanted to stay where they were because of the unknown and where they could have ended up. So we kept three patients that were pregnant, and they had extremely good outcomes. People die every day in hospitals, but no patient died in that period of time, which is pretty amazing," she said.

"By Tuesday, September 6, the water wasn't getting any higher," she said, "and in some places, it was actually going down, and people were being allowed to come in because until then, you couldn't come into the city at all." The B Team members were allowed to go or encouraged to go to Baton Rouge where Ochsner had a staging center and buses were escorted in. Anyone who was leaving would either drive behind the caravan or you could have gotten transportation. You could have taken the bus to Baton Rouge and had a family member pick you up.

"I had a car at the hospital, and I opted to just get in my car and go. And I took a friend of mine who is an adult single person who didn't have any family. She went with me to where my relatives were. That was Denham Springs right outside of Baton Rouge," said Jackie. "That was Tuesday, nine days after the Sunday we had arrived. You think I would've lost weight, but I don't think I did. I was so swollen. Even at that point I couldn't get my shoes on."

After days and days trapped in the hospital's disaster environment, many staff, including Jackie, reported feeling disoriented once they arrived at a safe place. "I was really so, so tired," she said. "Even though we had directions, for some reason, it was very hard to stay focused on directions. And at one point, I ended up like 30 miles away from where I should've been because I took a left and several rights or something foolish like that. It was amazing because it seemed like a science fiction movie when you went outside of the hospital, there was no life. There is no traffic. There seemed to be no dogs, no birds into the highway outside of the city."

She continued: "And then you felt like, why is that Burger King open? And why are all of these people normal after what we've just been through?" Jackie questioned. "The first thing I can remember that was really important was I went shopping. I didn't even go for food. I went and had my hair done and a manicure. Those were the things that I just had to get done. I looked awful, just awful. So then I felt better."

Jackie looked back on her Katrina experience at Ochsner with a kind of amazement. "When you decide to be a nurse, you know that you're working Christmas and Mardi Gras and things like that. You just know that that's the calling of being a nurse. But never in my wildest dreams did I ever think that I would be in that situation. I can remember every June 1st or thereabouts, we would have a hurricane kick-off season. Safety and security showed movies of what happened at some of the hospitals that had bad storms and some of the devastation that they had. I felt like that was happening in our facility, that we were in the movie, and that others would be seeing it in years to come. Even the nurses that came in on some of the days that followed, you can't explain it to them. I don't know if our B Team could understand. It was hard to explain what really happened," she said.

"Even though there were so many things you might not want to ever remember about it, there were so many things you don't want to forget either," said Jackie. Soon after the hurricane was over, Jackie remembered getting a phone call from a nursing unit in Utah. "Unlike Ochsner, they were an OB unit, and they got about the same number of deliveries. They called and asked what they could do for us. And I told them that there was one thing they could do was they could send us chocolate. Because at that point, every time someone would leave the hospital or come back, it seemed like they would just bring chocolate. And they asked us did we have any nurses that lost everything." Jackie said, "yes, we had some that had water to the rooftop. There were many who lost a lot but there were those who lost everything."

The story repeats itself again and again. A brave nurse suffers greatly yet does not leave a patient. She continues to care for the patient until the next courageous nurse arrives. Another nominee for the title Angel of Katrina.

Lessons Learned at Ochsner

—The advance planning and lessons learned from a Pensacola hospital during a hurricane made all the difference in Ochsner surviving Hurricane Katrina.

—Ochsner staff could call a recording for updates about news, shifts, operations and follow-up.

—Ochsner staff could bring their families with suitcases and supplies for days. Pets were discouraged, but allowed if that kept a critical staffer from reporting to work.

—Nurses got territorial about where they slept after their 12-hour shifts. They would team up with someone on the other shift so mattresses and sofas could be used to sleep around the clock.

—When elevators failed, nurses and staff assembled a human chain in the stairwells to hand off meals that needed to go as high as the 11th floor.

—Ochsner did not have air conditioning, but every patient room had a fan.

—Ochsner generators were on the fifth floor, above flood waters. Many other New Orleans area hospitals had generators in the basement or first floor—and they flooded out soon.

—The maternity unit had a much-coveted washer and dryer. Garments, linen and sheets hung in the operating room to dry.

—Medical students serving their residency at Ochsner helped the medical staff and nurses by making the rounds with patients.

—So many incoming calls flooded the maternity ward that the unit needed two nurses to answer questions from nervous new moms or those expecting.

—The staff could e-mail their families and loved ones.

—Armed National Guardsmen patrolled the Ochsner campus when news or rumors of looting circulated.

—The center had water for washing machines, toilets and showers because it was served by its own well. Few other New Orleans hospitals had non-potable water supplies like this.

Chapter 9
Lambeth House Stood Tall and Strong

"I probably didn't know enough to be scared at the time: I didn't know what was going on with people downtown, the looting and shooting," Kyle recalled. The only news his staff received was from a battery-powered TV with no cable access. Mobile phones were dead, leaving Lambeth House survivors no real contact with the outside world. The levees on the Mississippi River across the street looked beautiful, but nobody had any news about the flooding or the levee failures. Unfortunately, his staff of nursing assistants and aids found out about the flooding soon enough.

"They learned the levees had broken," Kyle said, "and the floodgates were opened." A frenzied scramble ensued with anyone who owned a car moving it up to the nearby levee to avoid flooding, praying the levee would hold. "At that point some of the females started screaming, grabbing their kids, their families, running down the stairs and out the door, knocking over residents on the way," he remembered. Kyle asked that his name be changed for this story.

The calm voice of reason was useless. "You know we're a twelve-story building and we can go up," he calmly explained. "You're going to take your kids and your families out there in this water with all of these people trying to get out of the city right now. You're not going to make it."

Viewed from the crest of the levee, Lambeth House is a commanding presence on River Road. Compared to a typical Uptown New Orleans wooden home, Lambeth House is rock-solid. Constructed in 1989 it is 12 stories tall, and designed to withstand hurricane force winds. At this point of the Mississippi River, Lambeth House has a beautiful, clear, view nearly a mile across the river and several miles north and south. The levee is wide, stout and well maintained. A luxurious carpet of green slopes down to the river on one side of the levee and gently toward River Road on the other. The US Army Corps of Engineers apparently thought enough of the location to build their headquarters only a few blocks away.

The most advantageous feature of Lambeth House when Katrina devastated New Orleans was its location on the high ground across from the river. This afforded an easy and direct route for evacuation that was high above any previous flood level. While approximately 80 percent of New Orleans flooded after Katrina, Lambeth House was high and the land did not flood later.

Lambeth House was in such a safe location that members of the New Orleans Police Department, the Fire Department, FEMA and Homeland Security were temporarily stationed nearby.

All of the favorable characteristics of the building and its location seemed to make Lambeth House one of the safest places to ride out a fearsome hurricane like Katrina. But to cynical local observers who had seen hurricanes all of their lives there were some drawbacks. The property was rumored to be the former site of an Indian sacred ceremonial ground. In truth, several previous businesses and an upscale shopping center that were located on the site had failed. That old rumor was enough to send some residents packing. The crowd had a name for the location—*The Curse*.

Some residents were also skeptical of the terms "modern" and "built to withstand category three hurricanes" because they remembered the death and destruction inflicted by Hurricane Camille on the Mississippi Coast in 1969. So-called modern, hurricane resistant mansions, hotels, and apartments were blown away, leaving only concrete slabs. Camille's 22 foot storm surge lifted barges, shrimp boats, and even an ocean tanker right over the beachfront highway. Further frightening local observers as Katrina approached was the forecast of the NHC predicted a monstrous 28-foot storm surge roaring toward Louisiana and Mississippi coasts.

In 2005, Lambeth House consisted of a number of luxury independent residences on the upper floors, and a skilled nursing

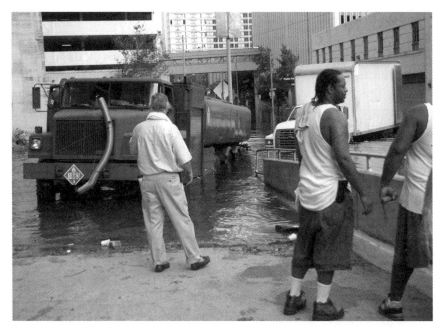

An Army fuel tanker delivers diesel to Charity and the VA Medical Center.

unit on the lower floors. As was typical when a hurricane threatened, before Katrina, many of the ambulatory patients evacuated themselves or were picked up by their families. On the Saturday before Katrina hit the coast of Louisiana Lambeth House had approximately 30 nursing patients staying in the building to ride out the storm and an unknown number of private residents.

✻✻✻✻✻

Kyle was an experienced RN devoted to the older residents. He had sandy-colored hair and worked with energy in caring for his patients. Kyle was also working on a master's degree to further his knowledge and professional potential. He was aware of the dangerous potential of Katrina and took the necessary steps to protect the patients and his staff. [1]

"We had a disaster plan," he remembered. "We brought our

immediate families with us, spouse and kids, to shelter at our facility because it's built to withstand a Category 3 hurricane." Lambeth House owned a 14-passenger bus that could have been used to evacuate residents, but the administrators of Lambeth decided to wait until a mandatory evacuation order was given. As Katrina moved through the Gulf of Mexico, state nursing home authorities reacted slowly, and like Lambeth, approximately 63 percent of the nursing homes in the area hit by Katrina decided not to evacuate.[2]

The order came. New Orleans Mayor Ray Nagin, and Gov. Kathleen Blanco declared a state of emergency and issued a voluntary evacuation Saturday at 1 p.m. At 9:30 a.m. the next morning, barely 19 hours before the monstrous hurricane struck the coast, Nagin announced a mandatory evacuation order.[3]

It way too late for over 100,000 residents and visitors to get out of town.

Lambeth House was like most of the area nursing homes that decided to shelter in place, and many simply did not receive word from state officials to leave town. Some nursing homes sitting on very high ground in sturdy buildings felt they were safe and beyond danger. A few other senior homes evacuated earlier in the week.

⨯⨯⨯⨯⨯

Nurses and the certified nursing assistants were in at 10 a.m. Sunday morning. The staffing plan was similar to the plans at hospitals and nursing facilities throughout the region. Nurses volunteered to come into work on the Ready Team, and a second group of nurses were the Recovery Team. By Sunday morning, the nurses who would stay during the hurricane had arrived. Everyone prepared for the storm.

"I had already ordered a ten-day supply of drugs for everybody plus food and water," Kyle said, "We were stocking up just in case." A week to ten-day supply of medications was the standard for hospitals and nursing homes that were too small to have an in-house pharmacy. The presence of pharmaceutical warehouses in nearby Jefferson Parish also gave a reassurance that medications could be quickly resupplied if necessary.

Nobody thought about the logistics of actually delivering the supplies to flooded hospitals, because hardly anyone believed the city would flood. For the moment the medication supply was acceptable, the disaster team was in place, and the staff went to bed for a restless sleep Sunday night aware that a monstrous storm was rolling out of the Gulf of Mexico heading for a collision with the Southeast Louisiana coast.

They did not sleep long or well.

At 6:10 a.m. the eye of the massive hurricane smashed the small fishing village of Buras with a 21-foot storm surge. Katrina gashed the levee of the Mississippi River, then headed due north. It rolled over the East Bank and made a beeline for the eastern edge of Orleans Parish. Sustained winds of well over 150 mph assaulted Lambeth House and driving rain hit full force on the upper floors.

"We thought the windows were going to blow in; it was blowing so hard that they were vibrating," Kyle said. Shattered windows and flying objects from the hurricane winds spurred the nurses. They hustled patients out of their rooms into an interior hallway, which was the standard practice. Medical devices, oxygen, and any other item the patients needed came with them. The roaring hurricane winds howled just a few feet away outside the hallway.

"There was no shame," Kyle said. "I mean, there was no privacy. You can't help it. We shut all the doors, but the storm just kept getting worse. The electrical power went out, and then the generator came on but only lasted a few minutes." In a strange twist of fate, the fan blades of the generator were turning against the wind. The generator overheated and shut down. The residents and staff were suddenly thrown into total darkness.

"You couldn't see your hand in front of your face," said Kyle. The staff had flashlights but they were conserving the batteries: so flashlights were only turned on when we were doing patient care or making rounds."

Lambeth House patients reacted well to the pounding winds and storm, "The residents were pretty good. You would think even the dementia patients would be excited, but they were fine. There was only one patient on life-support. We did have several people on oxygen," Kyle said, "In that regard, we were well prepared. I think we were left with about 24 out of 39 patients on our floor at that time."

The screaming winds told the residents that it was time to move out of their apartments into the hallways. Nobody had to tell them. Many had been avoiding the hurricanes all of their adult lives, so they simply moved chairs and treasured objects out into the safety of the hallways.

"I'd say it was about 10 a.m. Monday morning when the penthouse just disintegrated." French doors led out into the hallway where the residential section was located, and they imploded, according to Kyle and it took two people to hold the doors closed. "Downstairs on the first floor big, heavy sliding glass doors just blew away," Kyle said. On the first floor the storm crashed into the living room and the ceiling fell onto the lobby. In the other lobby, several men from the maintenance staff struggled to close the door and barricaded the furniture against another wall to keep the wind-driven water outside.

"The wind was blowing so hard right on the river. It was later learned some of the gusts were clocked at 235 miles an hour. The wind blew so hard, that the water was coming through the wall, the bricks, and into the building. Lambeth flooded on every floor." Kyle described how water went from one side of the building to the other, "It was coming out of the ceiling and out of the walls running across the floor."

The upper floors of Lambeth House were well above the treetops of Uptown New Orleans. The hurricane force winds above the trees had nothing to slow it down and winds well over Category 5 on the Saffir-Simpson scale smashed into the building. The building was buffeted by extreme winds on its upper floors and directly off the river on its lower floors, but its structure did not fail.

The hurricane-driven wind and rain forced the staff to evacuate the first floor and move the operations up to the second floor. Everyone—staff, nurses, maintenance men, cooks—scrambled upstairs where they huddled in the hallways with the families of the staff. They had never seen anything like this. Storm experience told the suffering people that the wailing wind and rain would be over in several long hours. For now, it was simply a mind-numbing experience.

The second floor was no secure haven from the onslaught. "On the second floor where I was," said Kyle, "we had one little area in the back that we couldn't close off. It opened onto the patio." First the canopy went, then the door shattered. Next the storm windows blew out on the second floor catwalk. Maintenance people had to pull doors out of storage and put them on crossways across the door and drill them into the walls." Recalling that scene, Kyle said, "That was really about the worst of it during the storm."

As the ordeal grinded on and Katrina roared past the city, the rain and wind slowly abated in the afternoon. The shrieking winds gradually changed into almost balmy gusts and slightly cloudy skies turned to sunshine later in the day. It was a brief moment of relief, but most of the residents and staff knew what would follow. Soon, the hot wet blanket of August heat and humidity returned and the temperatures got hot very quickly.

This started a different sort of suffering. Relived at one moment only to be faced with another trial at the next, the survivors glumly embraced a temporary—but false sense of security. They were in a news vacuum unaware of the unfolding drama. They were delighted to be alive, but soon to be hurled into a new horror.

Katrina's devastation started a cascade of ugly events in hospitals and nursing homes throughout the city. First the storm thrashed the buildings, then the power went dark, which caused failures of all modern systems—water, suction, laboratories, refrigeration, elevators, communications, lighting—that hospitals depended upon to provide services.

"At Lambeth House on Tuesday, the water pressure went out and we couldn't flush the toilets," Kyle recalled, "It was really starting to smell, and it was very hot." The telephone land line switching station was flooded. He was left with the only working cell phone in the building, and it only worked after a sweltering climb to the 12th floor roof in order to get a signal.

To further torture the survivors at Lambeth House, the Corps of Engineers had twelve vans in their parking lot with the capacity for 15 people each. Even one of the vans would have been a lifesaver. The Lambeth House manager asked if the staff could borrow one of the vans. He told the officials that patients were dying and they said, "Unless Homeland Security comes and authorizes the vans, we couldn't use them," reported Kyle.

"The dietary staff had one gas stove downstairs, and still cooking, but soon reached a point that they started making sandwiches," Kyle said. But after a number of the staff had departed, Kyle and his tiny group were overwhelmed with feeding the patients. The remaining family members were assigned work to do. "Of course, they complained," Kyle said, "but if they were going to stay there, they had to work."

The tropical temperature and extreme humidity forced the residents out in the hallways. In order to stay cool, the residents were stripped down to the bare minimum with no covers, with wet towels on them, and fans were plugged into the emergency outlets in an effort to keep them cool. The sweltering conditions added more stress for the weaker patients. It looked like the Lambeth House survivors were going to be there for a while. But the water in the street did not rise high enough to flood, much to the relief of everyone there.

In a stroke of good luck, the Lambeth House bus returned and evacuated a second busload of patients to St. James Place, a senior care center, in Baton Rouge. Many patients were carried down the stairs because the elevators had no power. They were hand carried down the stairs, some of them seven or eight floors.

Lessons Learned at Lambeth House

—Family members of staff and patients have been prohibited in new Joint Commission recommendations, but they proved to be a reassuring presence in Lambeth House.

—A van capable of carrying wheelchair or ambulatory patients is a huge asset.

—In a Category 3 hurricane, public utilities will fail. Plan for an alternative to power, communications, water, medications, and food. Lifesaving ventilators and other medical equipment needs reliable backup power mounted on the second floor or higher.

—Category 3 hurricane winds easily shattered all but the strongest doors, windows and openings. Stay away from all wall openings when the wind picks up speeds over 75 mph.

—A 10-day supply of medications and other medical supplies is mandatory.

A detachment of the New Orleans Police Department was stationed across the street from Lambeth, which was a designated refuge place because it is one of the highest points in the city and a hurricane proof building. Kyle said, "There were probably 12 policemen, a fire department detachment, and a couple of ambulance crews, but eventually they all left."

Wednesday dawned with the promise of another cloudless, sweltering day. The Lambeth House staff was waiting for its van to return. Lambeth had sent a couple of the sickest people out by commandeering large Cadillacs and Lincolns. They put patients in the back seats, and fought floods, traffic and refugees to Baton Rouge. The next morning, they ended up in a hospital. Those Lambeth House patients lived, but they came very close. "We loaded the people that we could, the wheelchair residents," Kyle said, "and the other residents in the back seat of my car. Then the housekeeper loaded everything in the front seat and a whole bunch of supplies in the back seat and in the trunk. We commandeered a bunch of vehicles, and we convoyed ourselves out."

The Lambeth House impromptu flotilla motored along on its own in a sea of refugees on River Road, trying to get through to Causeway Boulevard. Normally, one of the busiest intersections in the state of Louisiana, the cloverleaf at Causeway and Interstate 10 had been converted into a massive staging area. They could see thousands of people lined up by the glassy Galleria office building waiting for evacuation buses. Overhead dozens of helicopters were hovering to land with more refugees. Then the convoy met more water in their path to safety, but managed to plow through it.

"I was so happy when we got to St. James Place in Baton Rouge. We had an apartment that they let us use. We had to sleep on the floor, but they had the air conditioner going. I was happy to sleep on the floor as long as we had air conditioning."

"The facility in Baton Rouge had taken up a collection especially for the employees who lost everything. At that point everybody was tearful." After four days Kyle's friend Randy called on his cell phone. "I stepped out into the hallway, and there he was. He said, 'I'm here to rescue you.' I just lost it, I cried, I had a working cell phone, and my family was frantic, because they were watching the news. They were seeing what was going on. They wanted me to get out. But you know, I couldn't leave my patients."

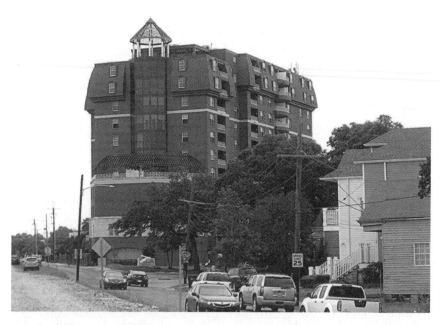

Lambeth House is on high ground across River Road from the Mississippi River and above uptown homes and businesses.

Chapter 10

The EOC in Baton Rouge: No Command, No Control

FEMA Director Michael Brown arrived in the emergency operations center in Baton Rouge. He seemed to be concerned about dinner reservations and his shirt supply rather than managing disaster response. He had the incredible lack of judgment to call Louisiana "dysfunctional" after it had been thoroughly trashed by the storm of the century.

The greatest natural disaster in the history of America was immediately magnified by the greatest manmade disaster in history. Over 90 percent of the telephone lines were out, cell phone towers were destroyed, and soon the failure of the levees would become obvious. Over 1,100 would die in the New Orleans area. Well over 80 percent of New Orleans would soon be inundated under a nasty cocktail of contaminated water that became more toxic as the days dragged by.[1]

And then Brown added that the EOC had no unity of command.[2] His previous career was managing horses.

Then President George W. Bush circled the destruction in Air Force One coming from a vacation from his Texas ranch. He did not land. Later that day one of the most hilarious wordsmiths in presidential history laid a memorable sobriquet on Brown.

"Brownie, you're doing a heckuva job," Bush told his FEMA director about the federal response to the Katrina disaster.

Brownie was gone ten days after the president's pat on the back for national TV. Brown was the first federal scapegoat for mismanaged response to Katrina. Bush would get his share of the blame. So would Gov. Kathleen Blanco and New Orleans Mayor Ray Nagin. That list would grow in the 10 years since Katrina.

Bill Lokey, the FEMA Federal Coordinating officer, had the good sense to remind everyone that the catastrophic nature of Hurricane Katrina was a primary factor in the EOC equation.[3]

Brown complained that he could not figure out who was in charge of the EOC.

"Just plain bull," fumed Jeff Smith, the Louisiana State Coordinating Officer.[4]

The command center was fully functional and it was always clear that Smith was in command of the EOC. Smith added if Brown really wanted to find the person in charge of the EOC, then all he had to do was look at Bill Lokey, and see that Smith was standing next to him. To prove his point, Smith produced a picture of him and Lokey conferring in the EOC during Katrina.[5]

✕✕✕✕✕

How do you get a straight answer from a bureaucrat? Should I go or should I stay?

Thinking quickly, Coletta Barrett broached the subject from a different viewpoint, "OK, let me ask you this question, 'I'm a CEO, I've got 1800 people in my facility, 40 of which are on life-support mechanisms, I've got no backup generator if this one gets wet and flooded. Now tell me, "do I stay or do I go?"'"

"I'd get the hell out!" the engineer said.

✕✕✕✕✕

How many had to get out? Coletta estimated between 3,000 to 4,000 from New Orleans hospitals she surveyed. She was low.

The actual number was 11,000 to 12,000 when you add all healthcare staff, families, caregivers and walk-in residents simply fleeing the floods.

And then 100,000 stranded residents on overpasses, roofs, the Superdome and any kind of high ground.

✕✕✕✕✕

As Hurricane Katrina moved north after shattering Louisiana and the Gulf Coast, the Emergency Operations Centers in Louisiana, Mississippi and Alabama tried to assess the destruction.

The true death toll will never be known, but the figure of about 1,100 for New Orleans is considered by many to be a very conservative estimate.

The State of Louisiana Emergency Operations Center (EOC) was located in Baton Rouge, about 80 miles of New Orleans. The most dangerous winds and rain passed it by, but it was critically impacted in ways that did not immediately become apparent.

Some of the most vital damage was the communication infrastructure in the coastal areas. The EOC simply could not talk to hundreds of the federal, state or local officials in the hardest-hit areas for several days.

Communication failure severely eroded EOC command-and-control that delayed relief efforts by days.

The New Orleans Police Department suffered a total collapse and lost its ability to maintain law and order.

Many New Orleans Fire Department stations flooded, damaging equipment and halting service.

The Louisiana National Guard combat units, stationed in the New Orleans area and Hammond and around the state had recently returned from Iraq only to be thrown into security and police actions in the city. Snipers, looters and residents who wanted out—and then back in.

Basic services such as water, sewerage, and power were knocked out for weeks. Mobile phone towers were down and so were landlines. Mail service? Forget about it for weeks. Only one New Orleans TV station was able to broadcast—from Baton Rouge. The *New Orleans Times-Picayune* produced a slimmed down edition at *The Courier* in Houma then from Mobile and reported through its Web site. But who could get the Internet in New Orleans without power or mobile connections? Ham radio operators helped with

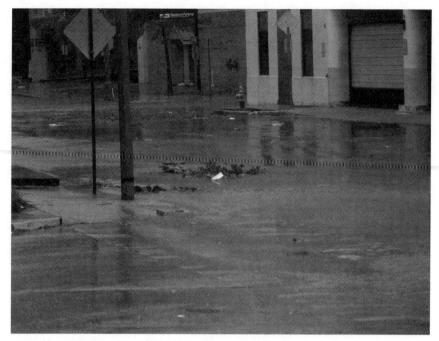

Canals and levees throughout the city failed early Monday morning and flushed millions of tons of water into the city, but the EOC in Baton Rouge would not learn of it until much later Monday evening.

their emergency networks. TV turned into talk radio, passing on news, debunking rumors and taking reports from listeners who had no electricity to watch the news.

Armed officers and Guardsmen limited even residents who could prove they lived in disaster neighborhoods.

Gas and ice were rare commodities throughout South Louisiana.

Hundreds lined up at fairgrounds, school yards and fields for commodity cheese blocks, bread, maybe some canned goods or MREs [Meals Ready to Eat]. Ice—if you were lucky.

✖✖✖✖✖

The EOC remained uninformed and powerless to help the survivors. No command, no control.

Designed for 150 to 200 emergency staff; the command center suddenly flooded with an estimated 750 to 1000 people. Why was Oprah there?

Many had good intentions, but more importantly had no business getting in the way of search-and-rescue missions and emergency response. Federal and state elected officials arrived with their associates to see the EOC in action. That only distracted professionals from their missions. Celebrities Oprah Winfrey and Sean Penn, among others, visited the EOC with media crews following them, adding to the confusion and distractions the staff would endure.[6]

Into this swirling mass of chaos and high anxiety stepped Coletta Barrett. She was a veteran, respected RN who rose through the nursing levels at Our Lady of the Lake Hospital in Baton Rouge, the state capital. She became an important part of the Louisiana Department of Health and Hospitals (DHH) section of the command center. Her responsibilities focused on hospitals in Southeast Louisiana including New Orleans.[7]

Coletta heard about the impending hurricane on Friday, August 27, 2005, at about 3 p.m. She knew something would need to be done at the EOC over the weekend. She sent out the Chief Executive Officers Alert to hospital executives with the hurricane checklist. The message said that the command center had not been activated at this point, but it could happen sometime over the weekend—so be prepared. Go over the checklist and make sure your facility is prepared.

She also sent out a notice to the hospital designated regional coordinators in all nine state DHH planning districts. The regional coordinators managed hospital information, response and readiness and other things such as the first volunteers and preparedness groups. She said, "If we get activated over the weekend, we'll notify you by e-mail and will set up our conference call schedule."

Saturday morning Coletta received a telephone call from Dr. Roseanne Pratt, the emergency preparedness contact at DHH. The state was activating the emergency operations center in Baton Rouge Coletta needed to begin her part of the emergency plan that afternoon, less than 48 hours before Katrina hit the Louisiana coast.

Coletta sent out emails to everyone saying the command center had been activated. The first teleconference was scheduled at 4 p.m. that afternoon. Conference calls started and continued every day at 10 a.m. and at 4 p.m. and would go on for the next week.

It did not look good for Louisiana and the hospitals she covered, she thought.

Coletta's role was to evaluate the hospitals, determine which areas needed staffing and then tell DHH where people were needed.

The conversations were frustrating. Coletta kept telling people who wanted to volunteer, "Great, we need you in Lafayette, or great we need you in Monroe, or we need you in Alexandria." Many of the volunteers wanted to go where they were not needed. No one was needed in New Orleans for medical support—but the city was the most requested by volunteers.

She called her friends and family, telling them, "You need to go ahead and get out of New Orleans." Leave quickly to avoid the heavy traffic. Major arteries like I-10, I-12, I-55 and I-59 would transform to one-way-out traffic contraflow to speed evacuation. Traffic would quickly crawl. She called close friends in New Orleans to tell them, "You guys need to leave and get away from the storm."

Some of her friends and family replied they were just going to stay. Many New Orleanians shared that attitude. "I was like, nahhh, you all need to go ahead and go!" Coletta said. She knew that in New Orleans many worried about the canals and levees failing.

✕✕✕✕✕

Coletta returned to the command center early Sunday morning but did not realize she was about to spend a grueling week working almost 24 hours a day. She didn't leave until the following Friday— when all the stricken hospitals had finally been evacuated.

Charity Hospital was one of the first New Orleans area hospitals to report information with an 800 MHz radio Although the radio is known for its range and reliability, some hospitals did not have the radio and some radios didn't work.

"We didn't have our radio set up at the state command center, so we got one," Coletta said. "It was like, 'Wow, how do we make this thing work?' We had never been trained on what to do with it so it just kind of sat there."

Ochsner brought a few radios to the Office of Emergency Preparedness in New Orleans, but could never get them to work. Finally, the EOC gave Ochsner a hand-held 800 MHz radio. They could now talk from Ochsner to the OEP in New Orleans, the VA, and LSU.

※※※※※

The CEO of St. Charles Parish Hospital told Coletta, "You know, I think I'm going to go ahead and go. I've got my own ambulances." DeSoto Regional Hospital, in Mansfield, La., had an agreement to take the patients from St. Charles Parish, a high-income blue collar parish west of New Orleans with petro-chemical plants and distribution centers between Lake Pontchartrain and the Mississippi River. They left before the storm hit on Monday morning. "That was about the only hospital that we knew was actually moving their patients out away from the storm," Coletta said.

Much closer to the coast, but well west of the predicted storm impact was the small hospital Our Lady of the Sea in Galliano, a small community established by an Italian orange grower in the 1700s and later settled by French-speaking Cajuns.

The Lady of the Sea Hospital closed except for a nurse or two in the ER and a plant operator. They maintained the hospital until Katrina passed and the recovery team returned. Lady of the Sea moved patients out because of its long experience of preparing and enduring hurricanes. Coletta gathered their information so the command center would know where the evacuees went.

Monday, Katrina roared about 80 miles to the east of the EOC.

Although Baton Rouge was on the weak side of the storm, Katrina still strong enough to hit the capital city with tropical force winds and rain for three hours. Katrina bashed the Florida Parishes to the east much harder.

The early stages of the disaster slowly came into focus as damage and flooding reports trickled in from New Orleans. "We were able to talk to New Orleans, and there was some flooding that was occurring," Coletta said, "But we really didn't have a good handle on exactly what was or was not going on. We were able to talk to some hospitals—but not all." The EOC had not received any reports of the broken levees, the flooding that would soon cover 80 percent of New Orleans or any of the small river town below. The absence of communication would later prove stunning.

Later in the evening, the EOC received reports of the broken flood control system. Little of the news could be confirmed.

Coletta and her colleagues were tuned to information that they *could* confirm. She maintained a spreadsheet of all hospitals that had already failed or evacuated. She also needed to know how many patients, staff and families were in each center to give to the National Guard. The National Guard liaison in the EOC was informed verbally and a followed up by a hand-carried message.

✖✖✖✖✖

As Coletta gathered information she saw disaster.

At first all of the hospitals were coded yellow meaning they had power and supplies. When the generators failed and a hospital or healthcare center lost power, it moved to a red status, meaning evacuation.

A large desk in the EOC tracked critical status changes. For example, when Tulane lost power it moved up to a code red. They needed to get out.

Between 1 and 2 a.m. Tuesday morning, Jim Montgomery, the CEO at Tulane called Coletta. "We've got flooding in the street. We've heard that there are canal failures—breaks in the levees.

Can you give us an idea what's going on?"

No one at the EOC knew anything about the flooding. They had no firm information for Montgomery.

"Well, I've got about two inches before water takes over my generators," Montgomery said, "and I've got people, around half a dozen dialysis patients who need electricity—and we need to know what to do."

Coletta said she'd call him back.

Coletta said to the Army Corps of Engineers, "We've got a hospital CEO saying that they've got flooding going on. They have about two inches of water before their generators give out and they want to know what is happening. The water doesn't seem to be rising as fast as it was. Will they be okay?" she asked.

"I can't give you any information. I don't have it," said the engineer.

Thinking quickly, Coletta broached the subject from a different viewpoint, "OK, let me ask you this question, 'I'm a CEO, I've got 1800 people in my facility, 40 of which are on life-support mechanisms, I've got no backup generator if this one gets wet and flooded. Now tell me, "do I stay or do I go?"'"

"I'd get the hell out!" the engineer said.

Tulane's Montgomery heard the message loud and clear. He called his HCA corporate office in Nashville, and then called Acadian Ambulance Service and its Air Med Service who started evacuation of the most critical patients on Tuesday. Montgomery and Tulane could make this decision as a private hospital, but he would not be reimbursed by FEMA. Public hospitals would be reimbursed.

⁂⁂⁂⁂⁂

Coletta realized the enormity of the disaster that was unfolding. At Tuesday at 3:15 a.m. she requested a full-scale evacuation of the hospitals.

There was only one problem—and it was a monster.

The Coast Guard, the Louisiana Department of Wildlife and Fisheries, parish and local emergency responders and all of the other rescue volunteers were focused elsewhere.

They were concentrating on the survivors in the water, marooned in homes, and in far worse shape than the hospitals. Patients and people with a roof over their heads, water, and a meal were considered the lucky ones.

Coletta vividly remembered calling Jack Montesino, the Louisiana Hospital Association CEO, to tell him, "We're calling for a mass evacuation. This is not going to get any better. It's going to get worse. Generators are in danger of failing. We need to go ahead and do everything we can to get people out."

Tulane benefited from the resources of its owner, Hospital Corporation of America (HCA). CEO Jack Bovendor agreed with Montgomery's assessment and ordered the corporate office to contract Acadian helicopters that flew in to Tulane Medical Center to rescue the patients, staff, visitors, and their animals.

Tulane's good fortune proved to be a painful heartbreak to Charity staff. LSU staffers hand-bagged critical patients (forcing air into the lungs) on the roof of the parking lot at Tulane. They saw patients, families, and pets climbing into helicopters for evacuation from nearby Tulane.

Maybe others would come for Charity. Maybe not.

Charity Hospital staff and the command center did not know that most military helicopters, such as the National Guard, were not configured for patients. Coast Guard helicopters were equipped for lifesaving emergencies.

"The person on the other end of the line from Charity was yelling because helicopters were taking off with able-bodied people, animals and staff and they were still hand-bagging people on stretchers on top of the roof, yelling at me, 'Can't you fix this?'"

Corrine could not.

⌘⌘⌘⌘⌘

Wednesday dawned to a day of frantic chaos. New Orleans was flooding fast. The broken levee system was widely reported. Water from Lake Pontchartrain on the north side of New Orleans and Metairie would pour in for four days. Pumps failed. Toxic water had nowhere to go. It stayed for months.

Hospitals that lost emergency power first usually had generators in the flooded basement or first floor. Ochsner placed generators on the fifth floor. Ochsner had enough emergency power for health devices, computer systems, fans in every patient room—and power for a washer and dryer in the maternity ward.

Patients depended on electrical medical equipment such as ventilators, incubators, cardiac monitors, suction machines, and all of the laboratory testing machines.

⌘⌘⌘⌘⌘

Coletta estimated 3,000 to 4,000 patients needed to be evacuated from New Orleans-area hospitals.

The actual count turned out to be closer to 11,000 to 12,000. That counted patients, care givers, physicians, medical students, family members, people who sheltered, and all of those in the hospital. A massive airlift.

But it was secondary to the 100,000 people stranded in homes, rooftops and attics and high ground such as highway overpasses and taller commercial buildings throughout the city.

As the scope of the catastrophe rapidly mushroomed and anxiety ratcheted up, simple communication grew difficult for everyone.

Coletta recalled an exchange with the small hospital in Galliano.

"About the second time I called Our Lady of the Sea," she remembered, "The nurse was just fussing. She goes, 'we can't take anymore.'"

"Well, but you had nine beds," Corrine said, "and I've only sent you four patients."

"You sent me four ambulances," the nurse fumed.

"How did I send you four patients?" Corrine replied.

"Well, your definition and their definition are two different things," the nurse said.

"I got on the phone with Acadian Ambulance Service and they go, "if we're going to send ambulances, we're going to pack more than one in."

"Oh my God!"

The neonates or newborns, and children in New Orleans hospitals were some of the most fragile patients in the flooded hospitals. Children's Hospital had not evacuated due to their high elevation location. Children's sent a rescue team that used canoes through high water to University Hospital, picked up neonates in incubators, then paddled them out to fire trucks that could operate in high water. From there the fire trucks and the neonatal teams from Children's picked up the babies, and transported them to Children's Hospital. It was a daring rescue, but without reliable power, there were few options.

Coletta reported, "Between Woman's Hospital in Baton Rouge and Lafayette General Hospital with their neonatal unit, they were able to handle flights out of New Orleans on helicopters to get all the kids out and the neonates evacuated. That was a very controlled evacuation. We knew exactly where the kids went," she recalled.

Their parents were another problem.

The mothers and fathers of the evacuated babies faced a tougher trip than their kids. The helicopters that were configured for the neonates barely had room for the traveling incubator and a nurse. Adults were out of the question. New parents are nervous enough. Anxiety suddenly intensified by the sight of their babies flying out of sight in a helicopter.

"It was a bit disconcerting, but they always knew where the kid was going," Coletta said. "We knew exactly where the kids were and knew the status. We didn't know where the parents were, but the parents knew where the children were, and they could find them."

The neonatal evacuation worked so well that it became a

recommendation to replicate: a separate evacuation process for the neonates and children. However, the baby evacuation was not perfect. The Well Baby Nursery at University Hospital, part of Charity Hospital, was somehow forgotten. The babies did not get out until Friday. Gunshots erupted. The babies had been scheduled to be rescued, but gunshots were heard, and the rescue mission was canceled.

Coletta next focused on Chalmette. It's a small community founded in the 1700s by a Quebec plantation owner downriver from New Orleans. Chalmette is known for many things, including the Battle of New Orleans in 1815. And losing about 46 percent of its population in the Katrina decade 2000 to 2010.

The EOC had not talked with Chalmette Medical Center. All of the patients and the staff were up on the roof and were waiting to be rescued. That's all the command center knew. There was no helipad. The hospital roof was not strong enough for a helicopter, so they were going to be boated out.

Chalmette topography posed problems for evacuation by boat. The land was very low; almost sea level and a system of levees and land structures made boat evacuations difficult. Chalmette and St. Bernard Parish were populated by people who made their living from the sea and many others who were accustomed to operating small boats in tight situations. Shrimpers, fishermen, oystermen. By Wednesday, volunteers in boats were rescuing the people off the roof at Chalmette Medical Center and then ferrying them out to a staging area on higher ground.

In rescue terms, a staging area out of harm's way is called a "Lily Pad." From the Lily Pad the residents were moved to higher ground or safer areas. From there they were moved to the search-and-rescue base of operations. Finally, they were bused or flown to Baton Rouge, Thibodaux or Houston.

⁂⁂⁂⁂⁂

The command center had to depend on politicians for

communication in areas like Chalmette where no direct contact was available. The EOC had communication with the parent company of Chalmette Medical Center, Universal Health Services, whose managers shared information they thought was accurate.

By Wednesday, the patients from Chalmette hospital were moved to the parish jail. They were all out of the hospital. But the EOC received reports that some patients remained in the hospital.

"No, I got them all out," State Sen. Walter Boasso said, "They are all out."

"Early Thursday morning we got a ham radio message saying that there were still people on the rooftop at Chalmette," Coletta said. "We had to track down Sen. Boasso again and say, Buddy, you ain't got them all out, You still got some up there."

"He was mortified because he kept telling everybody, 'They're all out.' And one of the people left behind on the roof was a relative. So he hasn't heard the end of that one," Coletta recalled.

✕✕✕✕✕

Chalmette Medical Center's sister, Pendleton Memorial Methodist Hospital, was also owned by Universal Health Services. Pendleton had marginally better communications.

The command center could talk to someone at the company: their lobbyist. The lobbyist reached the EOC to request security and report that Pendleton had lost its generators.

Katrina struck the hospital, and with so much devastation around them, residents were seeking shelter of last resort. Pendleton couldn't secure the building. They asked for the National Guard. Coletta asked Guardsmen to fly to Pendleton.

✕✕✕✕✕

"So here we are rescuing people off bridge tops, getting people out of harm's way, and the whole air space shuts down so Air

Force One can come in. They promised us they would not shut
down search-and-rescue when the president came through. They
promised but didn't deliver. Sen. Landrieu's office called and
confirmed that they would not shut air space down when Air Force
One came in through New Orleans, but they shut it down anyway,"
Coletta fumed.

"The New Orleans mayor was there, too. He was at the New
Orleans OEP. There was an EOC in each region like we have in
Baton Rouge," she explained. "However, they called theirs OEP,
Office of Emergency Preparedness. That is how you differentiate
the OEP from the EOC. There was a New Orleans emergency
operations center at City Hall."

Coletta excused herself, found an empty office, and just cried.

"You just do the best you can," one of the EOC staff told her.
"He gave me a big hug and said, 'Now is not the time to lose it.
You've got to get it back under control because too many depend
upon you.'"

She composed herself and returned to the command center.

⨯⨯⨯⨯⨯

By Thursday evening, confusion, exhaustion and frayed nerves
had reached a high water mark in the emergency system. As
survivors fled to Baton Rouge for aid, the hospitals quickly became
overwhelmed.

Some survivors were shunted to Earl K. Long Hospital in Baton
Rouge, much to the chagrin of the receiving doctor.

"Don't you be sending me any people in buses," the doctor at
Earl K. Long yelled at Coletta.

"Can you take care of them?" Coletta asked.

"That's not the issue. Don't send us people in buses," the doctor
yelled.

"Can you take care of them?"

"I came back because it was a doctor who is a pediatric

pulmonologist there and he was the doctor in charge for that day trying to get the hospital set up. He was yelling at me about, you know, you don't know anything about intake control and you don't know blah blah blah. I just kept asking, can you take care of the patients? He finally said yeah then he hung up. I was like, just get it done, take care of the people," she said.

"Six months later at a presentation at East Jefferson Hospital for the neonatal commission this doctor gets up. I was looking at him and thought *that is who yelled at me*. When he got finished, I introduced myself to him, and I told him who I was and that I worked at Our Lady of the Lake. And he goes, 'Can you top that?'

"You remember Thursday, 3 a.m., yelling at somebody at EOC because they don't know what the hell they're doing and they were sending people in buses?" I said. That was me."

"Oh," he said.

"Nice to know you, Dr. Asshole."

"Ah, ah, ah, ah,"

"'You're very friendly,'" I said "'but now when I see you in the hall, I'm going to call you Dr. A, because you're Dr. Asshole to me.' He was just mortified!"

"In that situation, everyone was stressed. But what you really saw, what I saw in the research that I did later, it was about decision-making under stress and how people make decisions during crisis. It was really very interesting because you go back to your basic, core competencies such as your ethical framework, a framework for decision-making, because that's where you have to filter everything else. It was just hard for us to make decisions, and it was very interesting to see how people grew in diversity, you know, and were very, very good at decision making," she said.

"You'll never have all the information you need to make a decision," she said thoughtfully. "You make the best decision you can with what's available and then you move forward. You know that it was just people who couldn't make a decision and became ineffective. Then it was time to move them to the side and I was okay. We had some of that happening due to stress. It may be the wrong decision, but no decision was worse. At that point in time, you simply had to keep going and do it. It was really interesting, watching how different people responded under stress," she recalled.

※※※※※

One of the most frustrating limitations at the command center was air logistics.

Hospitals waited for airlifts. Choppers deposited evacuees at nearby Louis Armstrong New Orleans Airport. Medical treatment was limited there as the staging area swelled over 5,000.

Baton Rouge hospitals were flooded by "bus people."

Meanwhile, more than 300 beds in Shreveport and almost 300 in Monroe were available and waiting for patients, but the helicopters did not have the range to fly from New Orleans to those beds.

It was too far. The evacuation helicopters could fly only about 150 nautical miles. By air it is around 250. The only thing that could have been done was to shuttle people out of New Orleans to Alexandria. Then use Alexandria as a base of operations, and then send them out to Shreveport and Monroe.

※※※※※

"Katrina was the very first time that the hospital portion of the National Disaster Medical System had ever been activated. We didn't know where the patients were going to go when they left the airport. They would tell us 'Okay, we're going to go to Shreveport, and we'd go, okay, we will go to Shreveport.' So we're thinking they're going to go to Shreveport then Shreveport calls and says 'we're still waiting and it's now two and a half hours later. We're still waiting,'"

"When the EOC contacted the airport in New Orleans, they were told, 'Oh no, that plane went to Austin. Or, oh no, that plane went to Birmingham. Or, oh no, that plane went to Nashville.' We had so many false starts of them showing up, getting the ambulances lined up at the airport, getting people at the airport ready to triage and disburse, and nobody showed up. I mean that happened at least three, maybe four times up in the Shreveport area. It happened a couple of times in Monroe. And it was really very disturbing," Coletta said.

While the search-and-rescue operations continued, the hospitals needed supplies to maintain ongoing operations. The Louisiana Hospital Association staff had activated a command-and-control center at their Baton Rouge office, staffed 20 hours a day for the first 10 days.

The LHA communicated with other hospitals around the disaster areas to find out what supplies they needed. The New Orleans airport was shut down. Many hospitals did not have three to five days of medical supplies on hand because the current supply process is just-in-time inventory. Medical supplies are used and replaced the next day because it's just more cost-efficient. As hospital margins shrank, managers had to find ways to creatively reduce costs.

"We were focused on search-and-rescue. We had to turn to the LHA to do business maintenance and get the supply chain going and help hospitals that have been evacuated begin to communicate with their staff, patients, records, and that kind of information. We turned to the LHA and said, 'you guys handle that; we'll do search-and-rescue,'" Coletta said.

The American Hospital Association worked with the LHA in getting supplies into Jackson, Mississippi, and then getting them from Jackson to the area impacted by Katrina. The LHA was trying to find ways to get the supply chain restarted or vendors that were still available that you could connect to hospitals. For example, people needed oxygen. Supplies and equipment were destroyed.

Coletta couldn't worry about supplies at the EOC; she had much more serious challenges at hand.

Despite experience, training, and positive attitude, she was hard-pressed by the enormity of the disaster and the severely limited resources that confronted every hospital in the region. Like the thousands of federal, state, and local disaster workers, she tried to stay focused on the most critical needs of hospitals—and solve them.

"Hospitals have to exist on their own for 72 hours," Coletta said. "When we came on our mission, if there is a Cat III hurricane, which is what the Hurricane Pam exercise was all about, we knew that for the first three days search-and-rescue will be plucking people out of the water, taking people off rooftops, and rescuing people out of treetops. The mission of the hospitals was to survive for 72 hours, and we said 'Okay, fine. We're great.' But we had no concept of hand-bagging a patient for 24 hours."

"We figured hospitals and CEOs needed to have 72 hours worth of fuel for generators and if you don't have a holding tank, you need a contract with a fuel service to be able to deliver fuel to you," she explained. "Well, guess what? Fuel trucks don't go through water! All of the planning on paper did not prepare us for the magnitude of reality that people faced," she said.

Finally, on Friday, the staff, patients, and visitors of Charity Hospital were evacuated. Throughout the area that Coletta monitored for the EOC, her stranded patients were rescued. The intensity of the week was decreasing, and she could pack up her belongings and go home.

✖✖✖✖✖

Lessons Learned at the Command Center

—The new 800 MHz statewide radio network wasn't tested. Some hospitals did not have a working radio so they could communicate with responders and the command center. EOC staff had not tried out the new radios.

—Fuel trucks could not deliver to hospitals in flood waters.

—Helicopters that evacuated infants could carry a nurse but not anxious parents.

—Many evacuation helicopters had a range of 150 miles, so they could not bring patients and evacuees from New Orleans to Monroe and Shreveport, where nearly 600 hospitals beds were available.

—Many evacuation helicopters were not equipped to carry critically-ill patients and their life-support equipment.

—The Louisiana Hospital Association and the American Hospital Association tried to identify needs at each beleagued hospital. Supplies were staged in Jackson, Miss. And then moved into Louisiana.

—Hospitals like Pendleton called for National Guardsmen to help secure their building as residents in the area sought a shelter of last resort.

—The state command center was distracted by visitors such as Oprah Winfrey and Sean Penn and their media followers. The center, built for 150 to 200, sometimes swelled to 1,000.

—The National Disaster Medical System had not been tested until Katrina. Responders and the command center could not track, for example, where evacuees went after they landed at an airport or a city outside the disaster zone.

Chapter 11

The Joint Commission
Reacts Decisively

Here's what hospital execs and their nurses and doctors learned after three deadly hurricanes. These lessons are useful for every healthcare professional, doctor, EMT—and every consumer who turns to them for help in a disaster.

The year 2005 was a watershed year for hospital disasters. Three powerful hurricanes hit the Gulf Coast in August, September and October. Katrina smashed the New Orleans/Mississippi Gulf Coast region, devastating a region the size of Great Britain and stretching from Louisiana into Florida.

In September, Hurricane Rita plowed ashore near the Texas and Louisiana border, and extensively damaged Southeast Texas and Southwest Louisiana.

And on October 24, very late in the hurricane season, Hurricane Wilma devastated Florida.

Like Katrina, Wilma was a Category 3 storm that approached Florida from the south and surprised residents by maintaining its strength and a very high wind speed for the four hours it crossed the state from south to north. Perhaps Wilma's most dangerous characteristic was the extremely large eye—estimated at 55 to 65 miles wide. The strongest and most damaging winds of the storm are near the outside edge of the eye. Wilma's huge eye with its powerful winds affected almost all of southern Florida. The storm knocked down huge trees, blew down power lines, and caused broken water mains across 42 counties in southern Florida, affecting over 6 million people for 5 to 7 days. [1]

Emergency generators at 72 hospitals in South Florida came to life. Two hospital generators failed immediately, leaving the hospitals without power for hours.[2]

Many of the remaining generators would run out of fuel or fail later. Hospitals that did not have adequate water pressure for cooling towers and the heating, ventilation and air conditioning systems powered by generators simply went without air conditioning.

The loss of power also knocked out gas stations, clinics, pharmacies, and medical supply vendors who are critical for patients with medical problems. The hospital supply chain was interrupted. The medical supply companies that delivered consumable medical supplies, such as oxygen, quickly ran out of fuel to make deliveries to both hospitals and patients. The loss of power impacted patients who needed life-sustaining home medical devices and dialysis clinics. These two factors combined to send fragile patients to the barely functioning hospitals.

The Joint Commission, the guardian angel of healthcare, is a nonprofit organization that accredits and certifies more than 20,000 health care organizations and programs in the US. For over 60 years the Joint Commission has been accrediting hospitals, and now certifies approximately 77 percent of the hospitals nationwide. Its mission is, "to continuously improve health care for the public, in collaboration with other stakeholders, by evaluating health care organizations and inspiring them to excel in providing safe and effective care of the highest quality and value."[3]

Part of the strength of the Joint Commission is standard setting. Organizations that want to participate in the Medicare and Medicaid Services programs must be surveyed and approved by the commission or by state surveyors. The surveys take place every three years, and are unannounced. In June 2014, the Joint Commission was approved once more to accredit hospitals and healthcare organizations.[4]

The damage caused by Hurricane Wilma gave the Joint Commission a timely opportunity for a hurricane debriefing project, and in January 2006, the commission shared information at a conference. Attending the conference were hospital administrators and representatives of 30 hospitals from south Florida, representatives from the Florida Hospital Association, and the South Florida Hospital and Healthcare Association. Participants held a debriefing of Hurricane Wilma. They discussed the events that were positive for the hospitals, the negative elements, and steps they could take to improve their operations before the next hurricane season.

The commission summarized the lessons learned from Hurricane Wilma and featured them in the March 2006, issue of its publication *Joint Commission Perspectives*. Although the Wilma experience was the focus, the lessons applied to all hurricanes and many disasters.

The lessons raised in the conference were community planning, communication, patient care issues, transportation, security, utilities and facilities, and human resources and staffing. The commission pointed out that although these lessons were the result of a hurricane, other hospitals in different regions were susceptible to extreme events that could create similar problems.[5]

Certainly, healthcare organizations across the country could benefit from the hard lessons learned from Wilma about such events as power failures, supplying essential needs, and communications and transportation failures.

Community planning was the checklist item.[6]

The attendees viewed community planning in light of critical supplies for healthcare organizations such as oxygen, fuel, patient care items including blood, cash, and communication equipment that may be in short supply after a hurricane.

A second tier of critical supplies involved patients who needed prescriptions and medical supplies for home use, which would decrease their dependence on local hospitals in post storm situations. Although it seems obvious to the laymen that critical supplies should always be maintained in stock, many hospitals have chosen the "just in time" practice learned from the Japanese auto industry. The theory was designed to cut costs by keeping inventories low, saving storage space for more cash-productive activities, and maintaining a more productive cash management process. Hospitals that were pressed for space and cash flow held limited amounts of supplies on hand, and depended on the medical supplier to deliver as needed. After Wilma, hospital officials suggested stocking up on widely used supplies and vital prescriptions before the storm season and refilling supplies when they reached critical levels as a hurricane approached.[7]

Communication in every form was the second problem on the Hurricane Wilma conference checklist.[8]

During and after Wilma, all available forms of communication failed beyond the local counties or parishes. Attendees reported that electronic devices, including satellite phones, cell phones, VOIP, wireless, laptops, pagers, and the land lines failed to function after the storm.[9]

The vaunted 800 MHz radios that had been purchased by some hospitals could only reach hospitals and officials within the county, and users had difficulty reaching nearby counties.

The second communication problem that vexed hospitals after Wilma concerned incorrect media announcements that caused crowds to come to local hospitals for food, air conditioning, and shelter, when the hospitals only had supplies for patients, staff and family members.[10]

Another communication miscue involved pregnant patients who decided to ride out the storm at local hospitals—even though they were months away from delivery. A pregnancy hotline phone number set up for the pregnant mothers might be a solution to the problem.

Patient care topics for the conference mirrored many problems seen at South Louisiana hospitals during Katrina. For example, hospitals were concerned about taking care of patients when the hurricane made conditions in the hospital unsafe. An example was leaking windows and flying debris that forced staff to move patients away from windows to an inside hallway for safety. However, moving the patient limited the patient's access to oxygen lines inside the room and raised privacy concerns.

Hospitals could not discharge patients because it was not possible for them to receive durable medical equipment at home when vendors ran out of fuel for delivery vehicles.

On a more critical level, patients who needed dialysis treatments were forced to local emergency rooms, where power was available.

Beds filled quickly. Moreover, without a safe supply of water, dialysis was impossible.

Transportation for the hospitals was a huge problem for many different reasons. Ambulances were limited and were contracted for multiple hospitals in case of emergencies.

Ambulances are restricted from operating in winds over 45 mph in many states, which further narrowed their use in storms. The sustained high winds of dangerous hurricanes place a practical limit on the range and use of the ambulances and other emergency vehicles.[11]

Curfews imposed by law enforcement agencies to limit nighttime traffic had the unintended effect of preventing staff who lived in different counties from coming to work. They were forced to cross different curfews in different counties.[12]

Hospital staff and first responders were limited when power outages knocked out the gas pumps.

Security was important at front entrances, the ER, psychiatric wards and the nursery. Several hospitals wanted armed guards at the entrances to secure the center. And certain areas inside the hospital, such as the psychiatric wards and the newborn nursery, were units that hospital administrators identified as potential security concerns. Although it seems obvious that the Emergency Room entrance would be dominated by EMS staff, some hospitals had their security staff stationed at the ER entrance to control incoming traffic and to screen unwelcome visitors.[13]

During Katrina the loss of power destroyed the security locks on many New Orleans hospitals. Desperate residents flooded in simply for shelter and not necessarily for medical care. Already limited hospitals struggled with too many people. When electricity and generators failed, so did security systems.[14]

Security systems are useless without power: interior and exterior security system cameras, limited-access doors, power locks, card entrances and intercoms. "Once the electricity goes out, you're in the dark, so there's obviously a need for heightened security," said one executive.[15]

When the New Orleans Police Department was overwhelmed

in Katrina, the hospitals were faced with the probability of overcrowding when police could not come to their aid. During Katrina the loss of officers, material, and supplies was a critical blow to the New Orleans Police Department.

Almost all of the New Orleans and parish police stations, jails, and backup buildings were destroyed. The police department moved into the Hyatt Regency hotel during the Katrina, and later, to a cruise ship docked on the Mississippi River.[16]

When the power failed, so did many hospital systems. Since a large number of generators came online immediately, designated emergency wall outlets were available in most hospitals.

Heating, ventilation and air conditioning systems that require huge amounts of power were cut off. And since most of the generators were powered by diesel or gas fuel, the emergency power was limited by size of the fuel tanks. Daily operations were limited by the maintenance requirements of the individual generators. Only natural gas generators produced continuous power for an extended period of time, often over seven days.

Generators are a problem with almost as many negative features as advantages. The negative features revolve around the need for very large fuel tanks, sometimes as much as 10,000 gallons per generator. Locating large fuel tanks filled with highly-combustible fuel close to a hospital has troubled some experts.

Generators located in the basement or first floor guaranteed that the generator or its electrical switches would be flooded, thus disabling the entire electrical system. Most New Orleans hospitals saw their generators fail. Ochsner Medical Center placed its generators on the fifth floor.

Charity Hospital facility managers placed generators where the electrical cords could reach the vital nurseries, ventilators, and emergency medical equipment. When fuel became a problem, staff siphoned fuel out of nearby cars with surgical tubing. Some nicknamed it a "Mississippi credit card."

Many of the nurses who worked in the hospitals hit by Wilma had mobile phones that allowed them to talk to their families and

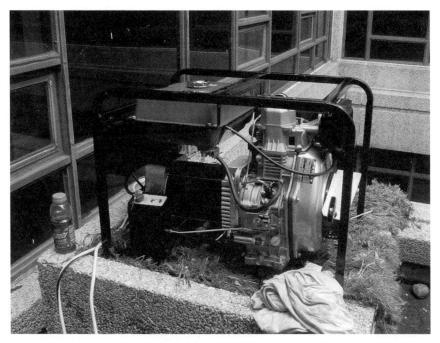

University Hospital facility managers worked around the problems by keeping about a dozen small portable generators going with hundreds of feet of extension cords.

the outside world. Since then, nurses have been discovering new electronic and solar power alternatives that help them survive storms, such as solar-powered phone rechargers, solar-powered flashlights and other hand-crank devices that provide light, power and radio without the weight and limitations of batteries.

The second most vital resource is water. Pure clean water is required for many lab tests and procedures, such as dialysis, as well as for hygiene, washing, food preparations, and everyday consumption, just to mention the obvious needs.

In a crisis, municipal water sources may fail or it can be compromised by water main breaks, as seen in Wilma and Katrina. Working in a non-air conditioned building doubles the amount of water consumed per person each day.

The back-up solution is to drill an artesian water and then treat the water. Ochsner had a well for non-potable water during Katrina. Most New Orleans hospitals did not. Florida hospitals had precious few wells when Katrina, Rita and Wilma struck in 2005.

Maintaining a vibrant staff is among the most vital issues learned from Hurricane Wilma.

It is well illustrated in every hurricane and every disaster that the staff is equally at the mercy of the elements of the event as everyone else. But the hospital staff has the responsibility of coming to work every shift with the energy and stamina to take care of all patients—even though they may have lost their homes and everything they hold dear in life.

Thus, the working philosophy of many hospitals was to welcome close family members. In practice, the staff often brought family, extended relatives, friends, and often their pets into the hospitals for the duration.

More people made planning emergency supplies harder. Conference participants concluded that guests should be limited to close family members to better plan logistics.[17]

Outside of the hospitals, the staff was faced with the same conditions that the entire region was living in at the time, including the mundane but important search for gasoline and food.

After Wilma, cash became vital because the loss of power rendered credit card machines, ATMs, fuel pumps and many other retail services inoperable. Some hospitals identified this possibility and paid employees in cash, which solved many problems for staff concerned with simple survival.[18]

Care and schooling of healthy children. Municipal sources of power and water closed all schools and daycare facilities, forcing hospitals to fill the gap by starting daycare centers.[19]

Lt. Gen. Russel L. Honore (US Army, Ret.) was the point man for the US Army Northern Command's response to Katrina.[20]

In his book *Survival* (2009) he recalls his leadership roles in hurricanes Katrina, Rita, and Wilma, and notes many similarities. He also wrote *Leadership* (2013) with more lessons learned.

The big exception was that Rita and Wilma surged ashore and

floodwaters drained quickly back into the sea, while Katrina roared ashore with a mighty storm surge that inundated the city, then took four months to be pumped out.[21]

The rescue missions for Rita and Wilma were not hampered by surrounding floodwaters. Some victims of Rita and Wilma could simply walk away or drive to find shelter. As many as 100,000 people remained in New Orleans during Katrina and many were trapped on roofs, attics and high ground. The Coast Guard and National Guard helicopter crews rescued thousands. Wildlife agents carried patients and nurses out in *bateau* boats and airboats.

Katrina floodwaters also stranded the staff, families, and patients in the different hospitals in the lower-lying areas of the city. This had profound consequences for the marooned populations of the hospitals. They were forced to survive on the materials and supplies from the original pre-storm emergency stockpile. The only cushion that the various hospitals had on hand was the individual supplies trucked into the hospitals by the staff and others. A further complication of the loss of power was that food that required refrigeration started to spoil. The flood had the triple effect of isolating the hospitals, preventing resupply, and destroying the means to maintain supplies within the hospitals.

Before 2005 over 85 percent of emergency hospital disasters were caused by events other than hurricanes. Fire, HazMat accidents, terrorist threats, floods, tornados, earthquakes, and other natural events have all caused hospital-wide emergencies.

In addition to direct causes of hospital closures, it is wise to consider disasters with mass casualties which suddenly overcome a hospital.

Hospitals and emergency clinics can be paralyzed by industrial plant accidents; large-scale car, train, or airplane accidents; and snowfall and waterfront disasters. All can cause a sudden surge in hospital admissions that can overwhelm the operations of emergency medical services.

Whether the disaster is internal or external, nurses must be aware of the basic steps to follow in disaster environments.

Staff nurses and unit managers offered excellent suggestions to prepare their unit's hurricanes.[22]

They replied that good housekeeping is an essential first step, and noted that they preferred a unit that was free of any nonessential items such as paperwork, supplies stacked in the hallways, and too many patient transport chairs or gurneys in the hallways. The availability of clear, spacious hallways is important for a number of reasons, and should be a standing order in all hospitals that is followed throughout the year. A free and easy entry and exit were just the start of a number of good housekeeping rules that the nurses preferred.

One summed up her experience by saying that a clean unit would leave no place for bugs or vermin to enjoy when patients were transferred out of the unit.[23]

The very important advance preparation technique is the strict management and control of HIPPA materials.[24]

Any item with a name, ID number, or any reference that can be used to identify a patient must be within the chart, properly secured, or destroyed.

Every medical device, disposable item, or material must be secured until it can be shredded or otherwise handled according to hospital policy.

Whether it is an X-ray or an arm band, it should be secured under lock and key or be a part of the medical record. Unsecured medical records are all potential federal violations.

Although all medical staff is trained and fully aware of the implications of HIPPA, visitors may not be aware of HIPPA and may not understand patient's right to privacy. This sounds obvious, but the explosion of mobile phones that can take pictures has caused a serious breach in privacy. Some naïve visitors may want to take pictures of loved ones and send them to friends and relatives. But once the pictures hit the Internet, the individual loses all control. The images are out in the public domain. Medical, nursing, support service staff, and students are all guilty of these infractions, perhaps because they think the images they send will not go beyond their friend's eyes. Too many pictures have found a way to the Internet resulting in HIPPA violations.

Although the importance of HIPPA material cannot be overestimated, the patient's chart must also be ready to move with the patient if an evacuation takes place.[25]

Ideally, the chart will contain the latest doctor's orders, test results, procedure results and any other information that is germane to the continuity of care for the patient. The most recent attending physician's name, contact number, and secondary contact number should be in the chart along with the doctor's transfer orders. It is a very handy safety precaution to place the chart in a large zip lock bag for protection when the patient is moved.

Almost as important as the chart to the patient's care is the safe transfer of an adequate supply of the correct medications needed by a patient. [26]

In advance of a storm, every patient should have a supply of medications for at least seven days, and preferably 30 days of medications. Although the pharmacy will not be happy with the cost of the meds, it is important to remember that the recent history of emergency patient transfers was chaotic.

Patients transferred into the makeshift hospital at the Pete Maravich Center and a field house at LSU in Baton Rouge were interned for an uncertain length of time. Some of them arrived with their prescribed medications, and many of them relied on a temporary pharmacy in an equipment room. Every medical staff person on site would have preferred to have the original prescription on a blister pack.

All meds that are transferred with the patient should be stored in a waterproof plastic sealable bag with the patient's name on each blister pack of medications.

Another advance preparation the unit nurse manager should take is a survey of the available utility sources on the unit.[27]

All the emergency power outlets that may be needed in a power outage must be clearly marked. All gas, electrical, and environmental controls should be located, identified, and their uses made known to the staff. If extension cords will be needed to connect critical medical devices to the emergency power outlets, then the nursing staff should have them on the unit. All battery-powered alarms, exit signs and emergency warning devices should be checked and new batteries installed on an annual basis. The date of the last check and battery replacement should be visible on the device.[28]

In the event of a foreseeable disaster or the beginning of the storm season, the nurse manager should keep as much disposable medical supplies as the unit can safely hold.[29]

It is much easier to have supplies on hand than to try to find something at the last moment. This holds true for disposable supplies for specialty medical equipment such as oxygen tanks, vent supplies, and for everyday supplies for typical patient needs. Getting supplies to the unit is much easier when they can be delivered by supply staff, than it is to attempt to send vital nursing staff after the power goes off. Conversely, all chemicals, gas containers, or cleaning supplies that could be dangerous should be under lock and key and known to the staff.[30]

A vital supply item is bottled water. If the municipal water supply or the hospital water supply is interrupted, sterile water or simply bottled water has so many uses that are irreplaceable for medical operations that nursing duties are very restricted without it. Part of the problem is that most nurses might think that a gallon a day should be fine for most patients, and that is true— until the air conditioning fails. Charity Hospital had tons of water strategically stored throughout the hospital. Demands grew for the water when the New Orleans municipal supply failed, and the lack of HVAC effectively doubled the amount used per person for drinking, bathing, and simple hygiene. Suddenly, the great need for pure, clean water became painfully clear to everyone.

The preparations should be completed at least 48 hours before a storm, but it is wise to finish the heavy movement of supplies when staff is plentiful and a deadline is not imminent. In the Congressional reports on Katrina, it was clear that hospital administrators had great difficulty deciding when to evacuate. The simple reason: hurricanes are unpredictable and speed up or slow down when approaching the coast. Therefore, it is wise to complete as many hurricane preparations as possible before any storm moves into the Gulf of Mexico.

As part of a staff exercise to prepare his officers to response in the event of a hurricane making landfall, Lt. Gen. Russel Honore routinely ordered his staff to start tracking the movement of hurricanes when they were identified and named.[31]

As the hurricane moved closer to a projected landfall, the staff had a list of prepared orders based on predicted storm movements to move personnel and equipment into staging areas on the left side of landfall—the weaker side of the storm—in order to be able to respond as quickly as possible. He contended that if a city or region was adequately prepared to confront the wind and damage, then the event was not a disaster.

All nurses must remember that patients are very vulnerable to outside wind, floods and temperature change. An important strategic responsibility for unit nurses is to anticipate such problems as broken glass and have a plan to protect the patient, especially if the patient requires a medical device that must be moved such as oxygen, a ventilator, or IV solutions. Moving a patient out of harm's way and into a clean, unobstructed hallway should be a basic solution.

Preparing the patients to evacuate should always be on the minds of the unit nurse. So many steps have to fall in place so quickly in the event of a move that everyone—not just the nurses—need to be aware of them. The unit itself should be ready to be secured quickly. All HIPPA materials need to be secured, and all of the computers, peripheral equipment, all portable medical devices, and telephones should be secured according to hospital protocols. A single phone should be left on a desk that is clearly visible so when staff return it is easy to find it if the power has not returned.

How many of these lessons so dearly learned are now actually applied? Since the Hurricane Wilma conference the Joint Commission has continuously issued updates in its advisories to healthcare institutions and will continue to be relentless in its review of hospital policy and readiness.

Chapter 12

Preparing Nurses for Disaster

What is the best way for nurses to prepare for disastrous events that will stress hospitals, clinics and senior care centers? How can healthcare staff prepare themselves and their families for long services during a disaster? And what training is available for nurses to work in extreme conditions?

This chapter is written for healthcare professionals, educators, and emergency responders. And patients and consumers who want information about dealing with disasters. It's written with questions and answers.

Nurses are the focus of these questions because they are the largest group of medical professionals to respond in a disaster—and nurses have a heritage of medical care in extreme conditions. In nursing education, they have learned and practiced the basic skills needed in patient surge events. RNs are the largest healthcare occupation, over 2.6 million are working in America, and about 60 percent of these nurses are working in hospitals, the Bureau of Labor Statistics tells us in 2012.[1]

It is clear that nurses will be increasingly faced with environmental conditions that are more likely to cause hospital overcrowding, a surge in patients, and staffing problems.

All that changed on September 11, 2001. The terrorist attacks on the World Trade Towers and the Pentagon brought emergency response into sharp focus for the nation.

The Center for Disease Control and Prevention (CDC), Federal Emergency Management Agency (FEMA), and the US Department of Homeland Security (DHS) became the vanguard of agencies responsible to organize and deploy professionals and sophisticated medical assets in times of national emergencies.

Who sets the standards for treating disaster victims?

Groups that set standards for treatment of disaster victims include private sector and professional organizations such as the American Nurses Association (ANA), Institute of Medicine, the Emergency Nurses Association (ENA), and the American Psychiatric Nurses Association (APNA).

In 2002 the ANA led professional nursing organizations with position papers and Web site information that gave nurses the paper "Registered Nurses' Rights and Responsibilities Related to Work Release During a Disaster." It's the fundamental primer for nurses to understand disaster relief work. It defines disasters, nurse rights, ethical issues, employer responsibilities, insurance coverage, national disaster policy, and the important legal issues from federal and state viewpoints. The great benefit of this paper is that most nurses have not considered these fundamental problems, and need to be grounded in these issues in order to make intelligent decisions.[2]

What about lessons learned for nurses from Katrina?

A year after the Katrina disaster, the ANA hosted a 2006 policy conference to develop guidelines for nursing in disasters. The conference was titled "Nursing Care in Life, Death and Disaster." Rebecca M. Patton, MSN, RN, then president of the ANA, aimed to engage the profession in three avenues. An expert panel was created to advise the ANA about policy involving standards of care, and to develop guidelines for nurses, institutions, and leaders for use in disaster care.

This conference was hosted for nursing professionals to review the guidelines and offer relevant feedback from nurses and others to the ANA. The final document was titled "Adapting Standards of Care under Extreme Conditions, Guidance for Professionals during Disaster, Pandemics, and Other Extreme Emergencies," published in March 2008. The authors planned a guide of practice for each health profession when a community emergency occurs.[3]

The authors also described the arena of the emergency as the site of a disastrous event, or a clinical facility, or at a secondary emergency treatment place. This could be a tornado, a chemical spill or school sniper massacre.

They warned that the guidelines are not a substitute for professional proficiency and are not a substitute for every professional and every institution to plan for emergency events.

The document is consistent with the basic principles of national response plans, but does not change the basic standards of practice, code of ethics, competence or professional values.

However, it notes that the local disaster environment is subject to change in relation to local or state laws that give the clinician protection in consideration of the conditions, for example, Good Samaritan laws. It also notes that extreme conditions force a shift to a utilitarian framework of treatment. Laws and regs change all the time that affect medical professionals. The Good Samaritan principles tend to protect nurses, doctors and emergency responders. Still, when disaster strikes, nurses should bend the rules to save lives. These suggestions and others are in the report.

The Standards of Care under Extreme Conditions sets some priorities in a disaster:

—maximizing worker and patient safety.

—maintaining airway and breathing, circulation and control of blood loss.

—and maintaining or establishing infection control."[4]

What else should nurses learn about disaster treatment?

After nurses orient themselves to these important position papers, and then study the basic information on the ANA Web site, the next step for the prospective volunteer nurse is to make a personal evaluation.

In a profession that is constantly confronting the reality of sickness and death, nurses must be honest in asking themselves seven important questions that will assist them in making realistic decisions:

—How involved in disaster response do you want to become?

—Are you interested in extensive training with the opportunity for frequent deployment?

—Are you more interested in only responding during a time of major national emergency?

—Do you have significant family responsibilities that will limit your ability to be deployed to another part of the country?

—Do you need to be paid during your deployment?

—Do you have portable liability insurance? Or, does the deploying system provide you with such coverage?

—Is your employer amenable to having you be deployed? Have you discussed with your employer the circumstance under which you will be available to be deployed?[5]

What should nurses consider about their families?

As Activation Team members, many nurses must consider their family members before they can make plans for themselves. Many times the nurse must stay days or a week at the hospital during a disaster.

So, nurses must consider their children, parents, brothers and sisters who may need special medical support and their living conditions.

At Charity Hospital in New Orleans, for example, so many immediate family members who came into the hospital strained the supply of food and water.

Should hospitals allow family members of medical and nursing staff to shelter there too?

Relatives should stay at another location, according to the Wilma debriefing held by the Joint Commission.

However, leaders at Ochsner and other hospitals found in the Katrina era that accepting family members and even pets helped make it easier for nurses and staff to volunteer for longer Activation Teams.

What does a nurse need to pack for extended duty?

After family considerations have been properly addressed, the nurse can think about preparing to function in the role of Activation Team member.

Perhaps the most important steps for the nurse to survive in the disaster is to protect basic needs by preparing a bag or backpack of items that are essential to personal life, such as medications, toiletries, extra clothes, hand sanitizer, first aid kit, extra glasses or contact lens, energy bars, solar powered flash light, solar or crank-powered radio, copies of important papers, comfortable shoes, and solar-powered cell phone charger.

Pack as much material as possible in plastic bags to protect other items from corrosive contents. It's handy to have a waterproof carrying bag with large shoulder straps or handles. It's easier to carry and could double as a personal floatation device.

Tell me about the national registry for nurses.

Once a nurse has decided to be an Activation Team member, then the next logical step is to reconsider their answers about their depth of involvement. The registry is important in planning for emergencies, and it must be stressed that a nurse should enroll in only one local, state or national system. Each nurse is counted as an asset in that system; therefore, an accurate assessment of medical resources would be defeated by duplicate enrollment in other systems.

The emergency registration program for nurses has a long name: The Emergency System for Advance Registration of Volunteer Health Professionals (ESAR-VHP)) It was created by the US Department of Health & Human Services to help states and territories build a national database about nurses for emergency responders.

It's an inventory about nurses to gather, verify, and categorize their licenses, skills, credentials, accreditations and privileges. It is a quick reference before a local, state, regional or national emergency.

It was created in response to the 9/11 terrorist attacks, when thousands of volunteers converged in New York City to provide medical help and recovery. New York authorities were overwhelmed and unable to distinguish between legitimate qualified professionals and unskilled volunteers who simply wanted to help. Historically, this confusing experience is common in a disaster. Sometimes qualified medical professionals have been angry and frustrated after being denied the opportunity to volunteer their services.

What does the registry try to do?

The nursing volunteer registration is designed to accomplish three goals.

—The first goal is to assist health professionals to accurately register their professional data consistently with local, state and federal laws so they can concentrate on helping others during the emergency.

—The second step is to help local health authorities find the most qualified volunteers during an emergency. The database provides the identities, licenses, and credentials of volunteers to help them make the best placement decisions.

—The final part of the mission is to help state coordinators in placing the best volunteers in the most suitable positions.[6]

A very important reason to enroll in a disaster registry is so that organizations can record the nurse's license, specialty, and experience that will be vital in any disaster response.

The nature of the experience and skills of nurses is an excellent planning factor in any large scale relief action and is one of the primary advantages of the disaster registry. It may also help with spontaneous volunteers. In the confusion and disintegration of an organized medical system, spontaneous volunteers who are not part of a registry are either underutilized or they may not have proper training and skills for the roles they are given. In either case, they are likely to be unhappy with what they try to do.

The Assistant Secretary for Preparedness and Response (ASPAR) helps each state and territory in creating a volunteer registration system that complies with national standards. Although each state has the flexibility to create a database that is effective for that state, ASPAR is the primary creator of guidelines, policy and requirements. The goal is a registration system consistent throughout the country.

How can nurses and healthcare professionals register?

The list of healthcare professions that may register for the

ESAR-VHP is lengthy, and some states may include professions that others do not.

Included on many lists are advance practice nurses, behavioral health professionals, cardiovascular technologists and technicians, dentists, emergency medical technicians (EMTs), paramedics, LPNs, lab technicians, lab technologists, pharmacists, physicians, physician assistants, radiologic technologists, RNs, respiratory therapists, and veterinarians. A volunteer may enroll online or by mail, as indicated on each state's Web site.

How are nurses protected by liability insurance or Good Samaritan laws?

An important consideration when making the decision to enroll in your state's ESAR program is the level of professional protection. In other words, does your state provide liability coverage for your actions as a nurse, and what state and/or national laws apply to your actions as a medical professional in an emergency. Many healthcare professionals purchase annual errors and omission insurance, and those policies should be consulted to confirm the type of situations that are covered.

Many states have enacted Good Samaritan statutes that may or may not protect healthcare professionals in emergency situations, and these should be mentioned in the state ESAR Web site.

What other ways can nurses volunteer?

On a local level of involvement, a nurse can volunteer for the Division of the Civilian Volunteer Medical Reserve Corps, based in the office of the US Surgeon General. It tries to engage volunteers to strengthen public health, emergency response and resiliency of a community to local disasters.[7]

The Medical Reserve Corps is a broad base of healthcare workers including physicians, nurses, pharmacists, dentists, veterinarians, epidemiologists, and other community members such as interpreters, chaplains, office workers, legal advisors, and other professions who can play important support roles.

The Surgeon General wants the MRC units to increase disease prevention, eliminate health disparities, and support public health preparedness locally.[8]

Medical Reserve Corps volunteers may help communities throughout the US. In 2004 the Southeast was battered by hurricanes and received support from MRC volunteers from around the country and locally. Volunteers assisted at local hospitals, helped in local shelters, and gave first aid to victims. Over 30 MRC units volunteered for more than two months and many more called in to help the responders.

How to find disaster training in the US.

Disaster training has never been easier to find, easier to take, and much of it is free.

Here are five authoritative sources: ANA, FEMA Emergency Management Training, Salvation Army Emergency Disaster Service Training Program, the National Center for Disaster Preparedness, and the Center for Disease Control.

The ANA has a number of nursing policy statements and guidelines about nursing in disasters that all nurses should read. The site also has continuing education units, or CEUs, about nursing ethics and other relevant topics.

FEMA offers independent study courses covering many types of disasters and is a gateway to information about government practices in the event of FEMA deployment. Many of these online courses are free and it is sometimes possible to earn college credit for the coursework.

The Salvation Army says that trained volunteers are the most effective volunteers, and their experts have provided disaster response and relief services across the nation and around the world for over 100 years. New volunteers may take an "Intro to Disaster Services" course and advanced students can take courses that are more specific such as "Psychological First Aid" and "Emotional and Spiritual Care in Disaster Operations." Check the schedule of training at Salvation Army locations nearby.

The National Center for Disaster Preparedness (NCDP) is perhaps the best bargain. Columbia University charges students thousands of dollars a year to attend, but offers NCDP courses for free through the very highly respected Mailman School of Public Health.

The Center for Disease Control and Prevention (CDC) is highly regarded as one of the most professional and respected government agencies. Its comprehensive Web site is filled with the best information on many diseases and their treatments, and they have the latest information on many disaster-related topics. Courses on a wide range of topics may be downloaded in either English or Spanish.

What about traditional healthcare education in the New Orleans region and South Louisiana?

Most colleges, community colleges and universities in Louisiana offer education and training in healthcare. Here are schools in South Louisiana.

Many expanded in the decade since Katrina. The Louisiana State Board of Nursing oversees these and all other programs from out-of-state institutions that may provide distance learning or satellite campuses.

—Baton Rouge Community College Division of Nursing and Allied Health

—Baton Rouge General Medical Center

—Delgado Community College Charity School of Nursing/Allied Health programs

—Dillard School of Nursing, New Orleans

—Grambling State University School of Nursing, Grambling

—Fletcher Technical Community College Nursing and Allied Health, Shriever

—Louisiana State University Health Sciences Center, School of Nursing, New Orleans

—LSU at Eunice, Division of Nursing and Allied Health

—Loyola University School of Nursing, New Orleans

—McNeese State University, College of Nursing, Lake Charles

—Northshore Technical Community College, Hammond

—Nunez Community College, Chalmette

—Qatar College of Pharmacy at Xavier University of Louisiana, New Orleans

—Nicholls State University, College of Nursing and Allied Health, Thibodaux
—Our Lady of Holy Cross College Department of Nursing and Allied Health, New Orleans
—Our Lady of the Lake College School of Nursing, Baton Rouge
—South Louisiana Community College School of Nursing, Lafayette
—Southern University School of Nursing, Baton Rouge
—Southeastern Louisiana University School of Nursing, Hammond
—Tulane University School of Medicine, New Orleans
—Joseph and Nancy Fall School of Nursing, William Carey University, Slidell
—University of Louisiana-Lafayette College of Nursing and Allied Health Professions
Source: Louisiana State Board of Nursing, May 2015

Nurses who prefer a more traditional university-based education have many choices across the country. Among the more advanced programs are the University of Tennessee at Knoxville, and the University of Texas at Austin. Online college courses are also available from a number of institutions and all are easily found with simple Web searches using the words disaster nursing education.

Tell me briefly about the history of nursing in disasters and combat.

RNs are blessed with a heritage of performing medical care in the environment of battlefield conditions. Florence Nightingale is well-known for her service to the British Army during the Crimean War during which she fought for cleanliness and comforted the wounded. Her most important contributions concerned the application of basic statistical analysis, infection control measures, and steps toward quality improvement procedures.

In the United States, Clara Barton volunteered to care for soldiers on the front lines during the Civil War, and later lobbied President Chester Arthur to form the American Red Cross. Although Americans could not conceive of another event like the Civil War, Barton argued that other crises would arise in the country requiring a large number of nurses who could assist in the recovery and treatment of injured civilians and military personnel.

Volunteer nurses assisted in the care of refugees and prisoners of the Spanish-American War. In World War I nurses volunteered to accompany the American Expeditionary Forces to Europe to assist in the care of the wounded.

In World War II nurses had become a formal part of the military, and the Cadet Nurse Corps was formed to quickly train professional nurses for the service. The war advanced the knowledge and skill of nurses by giving them experience in cutting edge medical procedures of the era, which translated to better trauma care and disease management when the nurses returned home. Tropical medicine advanced.

The Korean War introduced the need for rapid evacuation of the wounded during combat in extreme weather.

Medics in Vietnam built on lessons learned in Korea for evacuation by helicopter to field hospitals, base hospitals, hospital ships and specialized treatment in the Pacific or US. Treatment included trauma injury from mines, booby traps and chemical warfare, such as Agent Orange defoliant. PTSD grabbed more attention during this era than earlier wars.

The Gulf War brought more exposure to chemical warfare, pollution from burning oil wells and severe desert climate. PTSD injuries grew during this era, as well as during the wars in Iraq and Afghanistan. These wars saw severe trauma from IEDs, mines and hostile villages with no clear affiliation. And more PTSD.

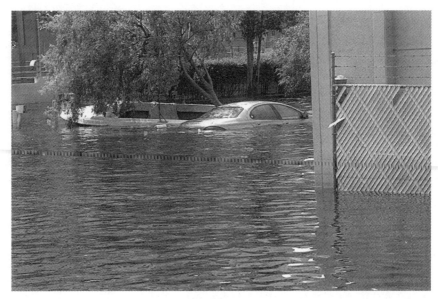

Floods from failed levees pour into New Orleans four days after Katrina struck.

Chapter 13

The Immediate and Long-Term Impact of the Katrina Disaster

One day before this book went to press in late May 2015 the *New York Times* published a story that confirmed the worst fears and accusations of many residents of South Louisiana. Almost 10 years after the monster Hurricane Katrina devastated Louisiana, the case remains open. Who is responsible?

Hundreds of thousands of residents may have a new avenue for redress. It seems that the efforts to pin the tail on the right donkey are ongoing.

"All I'm trying to do is set the record straight," said J. David Rogers, the leading author of the pending article for the peer-reviewed *Water Policy*. Rogers is the Chair of Geological Engineering at the Missouri University of Science and Technology.

Restitution of some kind may be on the horizon after a federal judge ruled in May 2015 that the federal government owed compensation to owners of property flooded by Katrina.

Professor Rogers states that earlier studies "may have been both historically and logically flawed."

The news story may take the old levee boards off the hook for the blame of the defective levees—but does not relieve the boards of criticism for conflicts in real estate, investments and corruption.

The US Army Corps of Engineers freely took the blame for the poor construction of the levees because they appeared to be immune from court action, but a new legal theory has changed that that long-held assumption that dates back to the tragic 1927 floods.

Judge Susan G. Braden, US Court of Federal Claims, accepted Professor Rogers's new legal theory for flood claims against the federal government.

The ruling will have significant consequences in future disasters.

✕✕✕✕✕

Hurricane Katrina could have been much worse—a common attitude of people not from here. The world looked at New Orleans with horror, pity, and misunderstanding. Starting with President George W. Bush, Michael Brown and FEMA. In Louisiana, the list started with New Orleans Mayor Ray Nagin and Gov. Kathleen Blanco.

The rest of the world had no idea of the deep love that natives and newcomers have for their city and its way of life. Was *joie de vivre* dead? Was the next Mardi Gras DOA? Could "the city that care forgot" live to care again?

Katrina's impact hit the pocketbooks of people across the country as the damage to the oil and gas industry caused the price of a gallon of gasoline to rocket from $3 to $5 in a short period of time after Katrina.[1]

Casualty insurance jumped. Flood insurance climbed beyond affordability—even with federal backing. Generators, lumber, chain saws and building materials were scarce all over the country. The price of flood insurance has doubled in the last five years even if a resident lives on land where flood insurance was not previously available.

For the nurses who were marooned in hospitals with no basic services, none of the hyperbole or economic impact mattered. They simply struggled to protect the lives of their patients.

Hurricane Katrina devastated the three pillars of protective services in New Orleans: the Police Department, Fire Department, and the healthcare system.

Almost immediately the city lost Pendleton Memorial Methodist Hospital, Chalmette General Hospital, and within 24 hours Lindy Boggs, Baptist, Charity, University hospitals, and the Veterans Administration Hospital would go under water and lose the most basic services.

Only Children's Hospital and Touro Infirmary survived on the East Bank of Orleans Parish, and they would be overwhelmed with refugees within hours. With dwindling city services both closed in the next week although the two hospitals could have remained open.

In Jefferson Parish, on the west side of Orleans Parish and on the weaker side of the hurricane, only St. Jude Hospital was flooded. Ochsner Medical Center and East Jefferson General Hospital and West Jefferson Medical Center were three of the largest hospitals in the metropolitan area to survive mostly intact.

More serious than the losses of brick and mortar facilities were the staggering losses of experienced staff and the world-class emergency room at Charity. The brave nurses, doctors and staff were scattered all over the country by FEMA and the worst luck. But many of them found their way home.

The "A Teams" or "Ready Teams" who staffed the hospitals after Katrina were many of the most experienced and skilled nurses in the region. The resilience of the nurses who ran the hospitals and

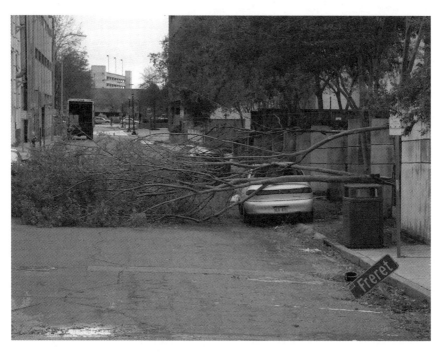

Hurricane Katrina flooded 80 percent of the city.

cared for patients was vastly underestimated.

In the worst natural and manmade disaster to strike the United States in its history, the nurses tenaciously plodded on.

Many of them slept on the floor and rested for 12 hours in indescribable heat, humidity, and utter stench, then arose to care for patients for another 12 hours, day after frustrating day. Often deprived of the most basic medical services, these brave souls soldiered on. Many others in the city deserted their duties and pleaded traumatic shock, ignorance, exhaustion, or incompetence. The courageous nurses simply found a way to care for their patients when everyone else struggled.

Throughout the interviews for this book, the theme repeated itself again and again, "no way would I ever leave a patient when they needed me, no way, as long as I was breathing, I would stay to the bitter end."[2]

⋇⋇⋇⋇⋇

After evacuation of Charity Hospital patients, these legendary nurses were promptly gathered up with the rest of the staff of the hospitals, and in the wisdom of FEMA, were scattered across the country. It is a testament to their commitment to serve and care for their patients that they returned to the city as soon as they could find a ride, a truck, or a plane.

Charity Hospital had one of the best and busiest hospital emergency rooms in the nation. It was run by the staff of the two medical schools, the LSU School of Medicine, and the Tulane University School of Medicine. The Level One Trauma Center at Charity was nationally-renowned for its treatment.

After Katrina, Charity suddenly had no place to open for business. That left the city with one small emergency room at Touro and a pediatric emergency room at Children's Hospital.

In the days after Katrina, many pitched in to repair and scour Charity Hospital from top to bottom. Residents of the two schools joined with the 82nd Airborne in cleaning up Charity's ER and

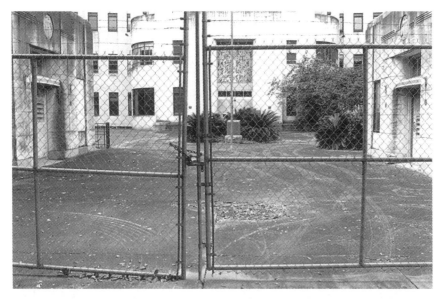

Inexplicably, the state refused to open Charity Hospital after Katrina.[3] Plot or plan? Ten years later, the carcass of Charity still sits empty on Tulane Avenue. Photo by John Batty.

basement. In the three weeks after Katrina, the first three floors of Charity were ready to open again.

The Charity ER began an odyssey of transformation from a MASH unit working out of the Ernest Morial New Orleans Convention Center, to a temporary ER in an abandoned shopping center, to a MASH unit working from a parking lot.

University Hospital's emergency room finally was restored and reopened almost a year after Katrina wrecked the city's hospitals.

✻✻✻✻✻

The nurses who were evacuated from the eight hospitals that were destroyed were bused to the Louis Armstrong New Orleans International Airport and other gathering points. And then flown to destinations west and north of the city due to the path of destruction on the east side of the city in Mississippi and Alabama.

As nurses and staff recovered their senses after their ordeal, they reconnected with relatives and friends across the country— but often outside of Louisiana.

After they found their way to back to more normal living conditions, they began to see the actual devastation reported in the media that they could not have seen in their darkened hospitals.

The city had flooded with a toxic soup that would kill people and animals and severely damage most of the homes and buildings it inundated. Fouled by dead bodies, dead fish, snakes, nutria and gators. Toxic with spilled chemicals, diesel, gasoline. E-coli bacteria was detected in the water Sept. 6 and the Center for Disease Control said five died from bacterial infections from the toxic water. Diseases from malaria to West Nile flu were feared. Mold blossomed within days where you could see it and within walls where you could not.

Disaster victims were faced with one of two options: if they had the money and insurance, they could return and rebuild. If not, it was time to start making a new plan for a new life. For some that did not include returning home to New Orleans.

Like the wandering Acadians, uprooted Louisiana residents established colonies. Houston, Dallas, Arkansas, Atlanta, Nashville, Baton Rouge, Shreveport, Jackson, the Florida Panhandle.

In the rush to evacuate nurses and staff from hospitals, the government plan was to airlift medical staff to cities and towns across America.

Just as the post-Katrina health needs surged in South Louisiana, medical professionals scattered. Many local hospital staff members stayed where they landed. Other staff members who lived outside of New Orleans or whose homes remained intact returned.

Hospital managers did not know how many nurses, physicians and support staff were available to come to work. And it was not clear that many of the nurses who evacuated would return. Most had evacuated and would not return for months.

How many nurses, doctors and healthcare workers would return to New Orleans? How soon? Nobody knew.

For many of the nurses who had evacuated into an area with a shortage of nurses, they found new and better jobs.

The decision was made easier with whatever insurance money came from their homes, and a new government program called the Road Home. The program gave the owners of flooded property the choice of a grant based on the pre-storm cash value of the property or a cash buyout. As of December 5, 2014 the program awarded 130,035 applicants $8.99 billion to start rebuilding their houses and their lives.[4]

In the decade since Katrina, news grew of Road Home mismanagement and improper use of grants by homeowners.

Nurses who had evacuated to cities that offered better jobs and better living conditions had an easy choice.

New Orleans area nurses who evacuated to Texas were faced with an interesting and lucrative set of choices. The city of Houston received residents from Louisiana in three different centers. The number of evacuees was estimated at nearly 25,000. Some were housed in the Houston Astrodome.

Responding to the sudden flood of potential new Texans—and a huge stress to city services—the city offered nurses, policemen and firemen a proposition that was hard to refuse. A new house, free utilities, and no taxes for one year if they decided to live and work in the city of Houston.[5]

At the end of a year, the nurses, policemen and firemen could leave or buy the property at below market rates if they wanted to stay in Texas.[6]

It was a very tempting offer for South Louisiana professionals who had just lost everything they owned.

✕✕✕✕✕

In the ten years since Katrina, every New Orleans hospital and clinic changed. Some closed: like Lindy Boggs Medical Center. Some disappeared: Big C. Huge new hospitals opened: University and the VA. They attracted a new bio-medical corridor along Canal Street. New community hospitals opened: St. Bernard Parish Hospital in Chalmette, marking its second anniversary in 2015 and built on a foundation of lessons learned from Katrina.

Consolidation continued: the two largest operators made deals. The St. Franciscan Missionaries of Our Lady Health System (Baton Rouge) and Ochsner Health System (New Orleans) each acquired or partnered with smaller hospitals.

The Medical Center of Louisiana, which was composed of University and Charity hospitals, has transformed. University has been completely renovated, and although much smaller than Charity, it has been adequate to serve the much smaller population of the city that dropped by half.

The Veterans Administration is completing a $625 million medical complex near the venerable old structures they will replace. It's over budget by 66 percent and more than 14 months late, with completion expected in 2016. It's called the Southeast Louisiana Veterans Health Care System.

The new complex will replace the current University Hospital campus and become the leading hospital for the city of New Orleans for decades to come.

Ochsner Baptist Medical Center resulted when Ochsner Health System bought Mercy Baptist Medical Center from Tenet Healthcare. After Katrina, the bottom floor flooded and so did generators in the basement. The hospital was closed in 2005-2006. It began as Southern Baptist Hospital in 1926. Ochsner said in 2006 it would buy Mercy Baptist, Kenner Regional Medical Center and Meadowcrest Hospital in Gretna. Ochsner Baptist opened a 12-bed ER in late 2009. In 2013, the hospital opened its $40 million women's pavilion center on the Napoleon Avenue campus.

The Lindy Boggs Medical Center has been purchased by St. Margaret's Daughters, a Catholic Church-affiliated nonprofit that operates two nursing homes in New Orleans.[7] Lindy Boggs Hospital, formerly known as Mercy Hospital, is a now-abandoned 187-bed acute care center formerly operated Tenet Healthcare. Mercy was founded in the 1920s. It merged with Southern Baptist

Hospital and operated together as Mercy-Baptist Medical Center until Tenet bought the hospital and renamed it for Lindy Boggs, the congresswoman and ambassador from New Orleans and widow of congressman Hale Boggs. The site overlooks Bayou St. John in Mid-City. When Katrina struck and the levees failed, Lindy Boggs Hospital was at full capacity with patients, some with critical organ transplants, and their families. The hospital evacuated.

The first phase of the opening will include a 116-bed nursing home, and later, doctors' offices, clinic spaces and a small hospital may be added later.

The Franciscan Missionaries of Our Lady Health System, based in Baton Rouge, is the second largest private hospital system in Louisiana after Ochsner Health System. Our Lady plans to manage an 80-bed hospital in the renovated Daughters of Charity Health Center in New Orleans East.[8]

They will be accompanied by the Daughters of Charity, an order of Catholic nuns, who have been nursing the sick and poor of Orleans Parish for almost 200 years.[9]

St. Bernard Parish Hospital in Chalmette marked its second anniversary as a community hospital in 2015. The parish-owned hospital serves a largely blue collar community of fishermen, port and plant workers among the hardest hit by Katrina because it is surrounded by the Mississippi River, bayous, levees and canals that connect with the Gulf. The 113,000 square foot hospital has 40 patient beds, an intensive care unit, 4 operating rooms, 2 endoscopy units, cardiac catheter lab, and a 10-bed ER. It has medical imaging, laboratory, in-house pharmacy, and rehabilitation services.

"We want to remain an independent hospital owned by the citizens of St. Bernard and to continue to work in partnership with Nunez Community College, LSU Medical Center and Tulane Medical Center. We are especially proud of our Telestroke program with Tulane Medical which has already helped save lives," said outgoing CEO Wayne Landry in February 2015. He was succeeded by Charlie Lindell.

Most hospitals in the New Orleans region and South Louisiana expanded and partnered in the decade since Katrina.

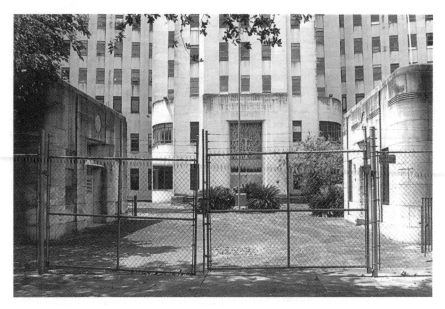

The massive art deco style hospital that was Charity is closed. The hospital that was once a haven to the sick and destitute, but also the training ground for generations of new doctors, now lies behind a security fence and is closed to the public. It is structurally sound according to engineering studies, but its future is unknown. Photo by John Batty.

North Oaks Health System in Hammond: expanded its ER and other services at the acute care hospital, which includes outpatient clinics, diagnostic and treatment centers, rehabilitation, a hospice agency, occupational health, outpatient testing. Formerly known as Seventh Ward General Hospital, it is taxpayer-funded and once staffed by nuns. Katrina's eye passed over the Northshore.

North Oaks-Livingston Parish Medical Complex: the taxpayer-owned hospital system based in Hammond for fifty years expanded to a campus along I-12 near Satsuma in central Livingston Parish and opened walk-in clinics in Walker. Cardiology, general surgery, ENT, primary care, rheumatology and urology.

St. Tammany Parish Hospital in Covington announced a partnership with Ochsner in 2015 and expanded its ER to 30 beds to serve specialized emergencies from children to geriatric. The expansion also included private rooms. It is a self-supporting, not-for-profit hospital that began in 1951. It expanded from 203 beds in 2008 to 223 then 232 by 2016 and is the largest hospital in St. Tammany Parish. Katrina's storm surge was up to seven feet along all 57 miles of the parish coastline, from Slidell to Mandeville and Madisonville.

Slidell Memorial Hospital and Ochsner Health System announced a strategic partnership in April 2015 that both sides said was neither an acquisition nor a purchase. Slidell Memorial is a 229-bed not-for-profit community hospital serving St. Tammany Parish and Pearl River County, Miss. since 1959. The Katrina storm surge extended six miles inland in Slidell and east St. Tammany Parish.

Baton Rouge General is a full-service community hospital with 591 beds on two campuses. It was flooded with patients during and after Katrina. In March 2015, the hospital closed ER services in Mid-City and expanded them at its Bluebonnet campus.

Our Lady of the Lake has expanded in Baton Rouge, Livingston Parish and New Orleans since Katrina. The Franciscan Missionaries of Our Lady Healthcare System includes an 800-bed Regional Medical Center; Children's Hospital; free-standing emergency room in Livingston Parish on I-12 not far from a new North Oaks clinic; outpatient imaging and surgery centers; Assumption Community Hospital; urgent care clinics; and Our Lady of the Lake College. The hospital began in 1923 as a 100-bed sanitarium in Baton Rouge and has grown to become one of the largest healthcare systems in Louisiana.

❇❇❇❇❇

Staff members are just as critical to the medical system as the buildings. As Katrina nurses and other medical staff fled the city, many had no idea when—or if—they would return.

John Jones, chief nursing officer of Charity and University, was one of the thousands of nurses rescued from a water-soaked hospital, and then trucked to the airport, then flown to San

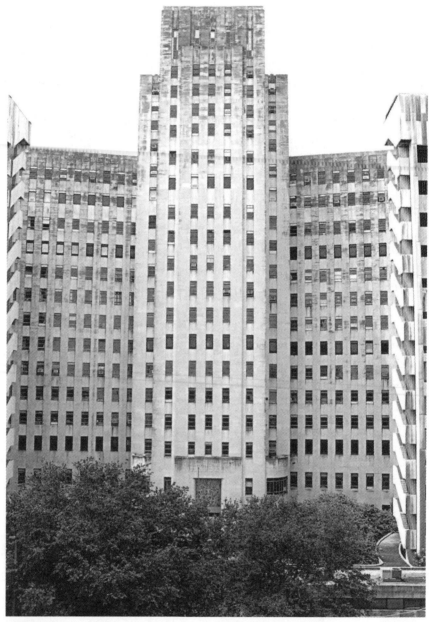

The state of Louisiana finally moved to ask for plans for the Charity campus and buildings in spring 2015—just months before the Veterans and University centers opened. Photo by John Batty.

Antonio. Although his home was high and dry after the Katrina, he endured a long return odyssey though Houston, Lake Charles, Baton Rouge, back to Houston, then Atlanta where his brother now lives. He has no doubt that nurses and hospital staff have endured Post Traumatic Stress Syndrome (PTSD) after days of surviving the hospital environments.

Katrina health professionals suffer PTSD twice as often as general public

The US Department of Veterans Affairs defines PTSD as a psychological condition affecting persons who have suffered traumatizing and life-threatening events such as accidents, terrorism, natural disasters and combat.[10]

This includes nurses, medical staff, first responders, and many Katrina survivors.

How to diagnose PTSD: The Diagnostic and Statistical Manual IV described six criteria that are present in the PTSD diagnosis.

Criterion A is the "actual or threatened death or serious injury, or threat to one's physical integrity,"[11]

Criterion B is termed intrusion, or the memory of the event which is experienced in flashbacks during the day or nightmares.

Criterion C is called avoidance and is described as avoiding triggers of the event, such as staying away from physical reminders of the event, emotional detachment from the event, or emotionally detached from friends or family.[12]

Criterion D is called hyper arousal in the form of insomnia, hypervigilence, irritability, and a sensitive startle reflex.[13]

Criterion E describes a time factor in terms of the previous symptoms being present 30 days after the initial event[14]

In addition to the six criteria, a number of interesting predisposing factors assist in the development of PTSD. The National Center for Posttraumatic Stress Disorder reports that 10 percent of women in the United States suffer from PTSD, and 5 percent of men are affected by the disorder.[15]

Katrina was the hurricane that came—and stayed. This prolonged problems with physical and mental health among survivors.

In other traumatic events, such as the Florida hurricanes in

2004-2005, the hurricanes came ashore, then the floodwaters drained back into the ocean and rivers, without lingering floods.

Katrina flooding continued for weeks.

Many nurses stuck working in the hospitals saw the media coverage and feared the loss of their families and their possessions.

About half of the nurses who worked during Katrina suffered some form of PTSD, according to Wendy Park, PhD. She found in a 2011 thesis exploring nurses' PTSD five years after Hurricane Katrina, that about one half of the nurses reported that they experienced psychological problems due to Katrina But the number who actually reported they were diagnosed with PTSD declined to less than 4 percent.[16]

Park attributed this disparity to reluctance among health care providers to seek treatment.[17]

Another explanation offered by Park was nurses most likely have met the criteria for the diagnosis, may have chosen not to participate due to these symptoms.

Osofsky, Osofsky, Arey, Kronenberg, Hansel, and Many released a 2011 study of first responders that found 25 percent had reported traumatic experiences. The study said 10 percent of the responders had significant levels of PTSD symptoms, depression, increased use of alcohol, and increased levels of conflict with a partner.[18]

A 2011 research report by McLaughlin, Berglund, Gruber, Kessler, Sampson, and Zaskavsky, estimated that over 29 percent of the respondents developed Katrina-related PTSD, but almost 40 percent of these respondents had recovered within 30 months after the disaster.[19]

These two studies indicate a level of PTSD that was at least twice the national average among men and women.

Charity's director of nursing John Jones said, "I was constantly watching my staff for signs of fatigue, and, well, we were all tired of the oppressive heat, the uncertainty of how long we would be there, and the stream of bad news. In the airport on the way out, I could see people who were there in body, but something was obviously missing from their appearance."[20]

As a manager who interacted closely with his staff and knew them well, Jones was concerned the staff was suffering from the initial stages of shock and PTSD.

Katrina did not end for months and months for many of its victims. Many woke up every day with the realization that the destruction was still around them, the devastation was freshly repeated, and the shock continued. For some persons who were fortunate enough to get out of the zone of total destruction, the pain went on for days. They were not home, they had no home to return to someday, and they faced a long period of recovery.

✕✕✕✕✕

The story of Hurricane Katrina is blighted by the failure of essential city services and manmade plans toppling like dominoes.

The city was stripped of its defenses.

Bodies were found trapped by floodwaters in their attic.

Businesses closed, looted and never reopened. Some were looters, some were residents just trying to survive. Some were cops on a mission.

Armed gangs ravaged parts of the Big Easy.

Mayor Ray Nagin mismanaged the crisis. In the decade since Katrina, he is serving a federal prison sentence for corruption.

When it came to the floods, residents spotted two scapegoats asleep at the switch.

Some commentators say it happened almost overnight, other observers cite the long incompetence of the New Orleans Levee Board and the US Army Corps of Engineers. They tell stories that the annual levee inspections had descended into an all-day party for the levee board members and inspectors participating in the job.

Critics point out that many levees were not finished in time for the hurricane season. Some were constructed of substandard materials. Even new flood control levees were found in 2014 to contain unacceptable fill material ranging from tires to shopping carts.

The public outcry about levee board mismanagement led to sweeping changes in the governing authority of the levee system in Louisiana. Members of the previous board were sometimes politically motivated and concerned with the development of casinos, marinas, restaurants and business opportunities. And new board members often knew little about flood protection or professional engineering. Although board members have been accused of doing nothing wrong in their stewardship of the levee system, they certainly did not serve many of the public responsibilities.

The negative public perception of the board performance was enough to vote a complete reorganization of the boards responsible for flood protection.

In 2006 the levee board reforms resulted in the creation of the Southeast Louisiana Flood Protection Authority with different boards for the East Bank and West Bank of the Mississippi River in Southeast Louisiana.[21]

The flood protection authorities require members to hold expert professional designations such as hydrologists or civil engineers, and only one local member per parish is allowed. For one of the rare instances in its 300-year history, New Orleans could boast that it was making positive municipal policy when it became among the first cities in the nation to name qualified professional experts to its levee board.

The catastrophic failure of the levees and subsequent flooding of the city have been estimated to have caused $90 billion to $120 billion in damages, and raised important questions about the construction and engineering of the levee system.[22]

The three parishes of Orleans, Jefferson and St. Bernard are at sea level or 10 to 12-feet above. Just barely—fifty-one percent of the land area. The rest of the land is 10 to 12 feet below sea level, according to a federal survey in 1999-2000. Therein lies the challenge.

To his credit, Lt. Gen. Carl A. Strock, PE, Chief of Engineers, USACE, requested an independent investigation of the construction and engineering of the Southeast Louisiana levee system.[23]

The prestigious professional American Society of Civil Engineers

(ASCE)) named a panel of respected experts in relevant fields to investigate the levee system. They called it the worst engineering disaster in US history.

Named ASCE External Review Panel, the report was entitled "The New Orleans Hurricane Protection System: What Went Wrong and Why," it described the event as "one of the nation's worst disasters ever" and levee failure as "breached because of a combination of unfortunate choices and decisions, made over many years, at almost all levels of responsibility."[24]

The report placed plenty of blame widely spread over many levels of government in the state and federal jurisdictions, and most commentators agreed with its findings.[25]

Two-thirds of the flooding in New Orleans could have been avoided if the levees had held, the engineering group said in 2007.

In March, 2012, the US Court of Appeals upheld a ruling finding the USACE responsible for the flooding the Lower Ninth Ward and St. Bernard Parish during Katrina due to its neglect to design and maintain the Mississippi River Gulf Outlet.[26]

Lessons Learned

—**Katrina flooding resulted from poor design** and the mismanagement of levees and flood control at every level of government, but primarily the US Army Corps of Engineers.

—**PTSD is at least twice as common among nurses** and healthcare staff who worked through Katrina than the general population.

—**St. Bernard Parish Hospital**, two years old in 2015, takes the lessons learned from Hurricane Katrina. It's been designed to withstand extreme weather and floods. Generators, diesel fuel tanks and operating systems are on the second floor, more than 25 feet above ground.

—**Prepare for total or major loss of power.** Although some generators came on as planned after the municipal power failed, the emergency generators were very limited in their capacity to supply power. Due to the enormous power requirement of elevators, air conditioning, refrigeration, and power security systems, most of the hospitals were suddenly thrown back into the 19th century of medical care and ceased to function as modern hospitals. Most of the generators survived the storm, but flooded electrical switching equipment or flooded fuel supplies rendered the generators inoperable.

—**Prepare for total loss of communications.** Well over 90 percent of the telephones, cell phone towers and switching stations were destroyed by wind or simply flooded. Only a handful of phone lines at any of the hospitals survived. Very few of the hospital staff were trained on the use of the 800 MHz emergency radios so that venue of communications was dead.

—**Prepare for total loss of municipal water supply and sanitation.** Although all hospitals had tons of bottled water, supplies were stressed by the very hot environment. Reliable potable running water was needed for laboratory tests, dialysis, sanitation, bathing, food preparation and laundry. Overflowing toilets gave way to portable toilets and five-gallon buckets for personal waste.

—**New Orleans was the medical center** of Louisiana, leaving the state with no potential location to evacuate patients. The day after the Katrina passed, almost all hospitals within 300 miles of Louisiana and Mississippi Gulf Coast were inundated with Katrina refugees and patients

—**As medical supplies started to run low** after three days in the heat and high water, resupply was difficult for the hospitals as well as the home-bound patients who needed oxygen and diabetic supplies.

Epilogue
10 Years After Katrina

Here are the real Angels of Katrina:

—nurses, doctors and staff who stayed in their hospitals;

—the US Coast Guard who plucked over 33,500 survivors out of the flooded city;

—the Louisiana Department of Wildlife and Fisheries agents who pulled thousands of victims out of the water in their airboats and jon boats;

—the New Orleans firemen and police officers, Louisiana State Police and sheriff's deputies who did not abandon their city;

—the Louisiana National Guard, many of whom had just returned from combat in Iraq;

—and the thousands of unnamed volunteers from across the nation came to New Orleans to help save a proud city.

In studying the thousands of pages of first-person accounts, government studies, professional opinions, and media analyses, the authors find that many people rose to the challenge and danger of Katrina to serve their fellow citizens in ways that no one could have foreseen.

While doing their basic lifesaving rescue work, they may have earned their angel wings.

And in the wake of the most damaging hurricane ever to strike the United States, more heroes came to New Orleans to help her natives and newcomers rebuild.

Thousands of volunteers from churches, charities and nonprofits across the land have come to help demolish and rebuild homes.

Actors, foreign governments, and thousands of citizens around the world have donated millions of dollars to the city for rebuilding everything imaginable.

Although the anemic FEMA and the federal response has been rightfully vilified, since then the government has poured billions of dollars into the city to rebuild hospitals, nursing schools, libraries, clinics, police stations, public parks, levees, highways and municipal infrastructure.

Ten years in, the city of New Orleans is in the middle of a building and rebirth of creative industries and professions never before seen in its history.

Business incubators like The Propeller and the Idea Village

Start-ups in healthcare, education, food services, marine and aquaculture, transportation, coastal management and preservation.

In the new Hollywood South, more films were shot in Louisiana than California or New York in 2014. With the Hollywood directors and A-list actors came the birth of support industries. Hollywood Trucks, catering, sound stages, studios in New Orleans, Baton Rouge and Shreveport. Angel funds for investors and directors and entrepreneurs.

The wonderful mix of Cajun, Creole, French, Italian, Vietnamese, Tex-Mex and Southern blue plate is rolling on with more restaurants than ever. Name a national dish and you'll probably find it at a hundred year old restaurant, a pop-up restaurant, po-boy shop or food truck.

Documentaries on Katrina and *Big Charity*. Action films based on the BP/Transocean disaster. And more reality shows based on Louisiana's swamps, gators, cypress trees, duck calls, the governor's wife. And more.

The transformed University Medical Center and the Southeast Louisiana Veterans Health Care System centers on Canal Street will incubate a new bio-medical research community that can only be imagined in 2015.

※※※※※

In the aftermath, it is clear that the critical failure of the levee system and flood control changed Hurricane Katrina from simply a very big, very bad hurricane. It became a manmade disaster. Parts of the disaster were forecast in vivid detail for emergency responders and healthcare leaders only a year before in the form of the Hurricane Pam exercise.

The US Army Corps of Engineers requested that the American Society of Civil Engineers focus the wisdom and experience of the most prestigious engineering organization in the country on the causes and failures of the levee system.

The group found plenty of blame to spread around the political leadership, the local levee boards, the state government, the Corps of Engineers, and many others.

The US House of Representatives and the US Senate both held extensive hearings on the tragedy including the local and state agencies, and the federal bureaucracies that were charged with protecting the public.

✕✕✕✕✕

And everyone who lived through the event has relived it, discussed it, ruminated about it, and kept the disaster alive in the public conversation. The Katrina experience is part of legend that is the city of New Orleans.

The importance of the event is reflected in the description of the lives and times of its citizens: all life is now divided in the public mind as the "before Katrina" time, and the "after Katrina" time. The great migration away from their beloved city had not been seen since the Dust Bowl migration during the 1930s.

And the numbers of troops deployed to the city and state have not been seen since the War Between the States.

✕✕✕✕✕

Katrina changed most every politician in Louisiana and every level of public agency—from mosquito control districts to parish governments, the Louisiana Legislature, governor, members of Congress, federal agencies right to the president of the United States.

One of the most extraordinary events of the change in the public mind is that it voted the levee board system of 12 local levee districts out of business. They voted to create a levee board for the East Bank and West Bank that was composed of professional engineers instead of politicians with questionable qualifications. It was a big "first" for Louisiana and the nation.

⨯⨯⨯⨯⨯

The public and private hospital system has risen from the mud of Katrina to a new age of healthcare in New Orleans and throughout South Louisiana. Almost all of the hospitals have been rebuilt or refocused to serve the public with the modern, state of the art practice.

Hospitals that Katrina did not close, Gov. Bobby Jindal closed in his quest to establish a Republican reputation for president.

The dismantling of the Louisiana Charity Hospital System was at the hands of Jindal—not Katrina. Landmark hospitals around the state disappeared. Earl K. Long in Baton Rouge. Big Charity, which Gov. Huey Long championed in the 1930s, never reopened after Katrina.

Public hospitals that largely served the poor were ordered closed, privatized or were absorbed into the LSU Healthcare System.

That happened in Independence, La. where Lallie Kemp Charity Hospital has served all comers, starting with the poor and uninsured since 1939. It's now Lallie Kemp Regional Medical Center, part of LSU Healthcare. In 2013, the Jindal administration cut the staff from around 415 by nearly a hundred. The surviving staff suddenly lost specialties—and gained more state prisoner patients who displaced civilian patients who needed cancer and dialysis treatment. Lallie Kemp had been a teaching hospital for over a dozen medical schools and nursing schools. Much of that opportunity disappeared too with the Jindal cuts.

Venerable old Charity Hospital lies dormant on Tulane Avenue, its future uncertain.

Only a few blocks away, the $1.1 billion University Medical Center missed its opening date. Lack of money was blamed. Then the Louisiana Legislature voted to fund it in June 2015.

Louisiana Treasurer John Kennedy suggested otherwise in an op-ed column March 16, 2015 in the *New Orleans Times-Picayune*. "I did not support spending $1.1 billion on a new facility. The old Big Charity is a beautiful, art deco building and could have been renovated for half the price of a new one. US Sen. David Vitter, then House Speaker Jim Tucker and I offered another proposal, saving hundreds of millions of dollars, to purchase Tulane Hospital and then build a new hospital with a smaller footprint. We were out-voted. Now University Medical Center is built. We invested more than a billion dollars of Louisiana and American taxpayer money into the facility. We built it. We've got to open it, and we've got to make it work. Failure is not an option."

Nearby, the new Southeast Louisiana Veterans Health Care Center expects to open in 2016, already 14 months overdue and 66 percent over its original budget.

And this time the generators and the electrical switching equipment will be located above the flood plain.

⁂⁂⁂⁂⁂

The angels who were scattered across the country have returned. Most of their patients have found their way home, and the city is rising out of the muck in a new, exciting version of its old self. The shake, rattle and roll of the music is back, and young new musicians are filling the air with their sounds.

The angels who were willing to give their lives to protect and save others are back—or planning to return one day. Maybe they were born to be the persons who care for others. Perhaps their personalities are encoded in their DNA.

Maybe they were there at the right place and the right time. They stepped up.

To the doctors and medical staff who saw these nurses in action, they know an angel when they see one.

Southeast Louisiana Veterans Healthcare System New Orleans

What's in a name: Nicknamed Project Legacy, the name chosen from among 85 nominees.

Original budget: $625 million. In mid-2015, the center was 66 percent over that budget and 14 months late.

Leader: Fernando Oscar Rivera, director and CEO, who replaced Julie Catelier who retired in 2014.

Construction: Clark/McCarthy Healthcare Partners.

Location: Bounded by Canal Street, S. Rocheblave Street, S. Galvez Street and Tulane Avenue—blocks north from the old VA Medical Center New Orleans. It will be near the new University Medical Center.

By the numbers: Construction designed to withstand a Category 3 hurricane. Rainwater storage, storage for over 300,000 gallons of fuel, and a 6,000 square foot emergency warehouse. The center is huge, stretching from Canal Street to Tulane Avenue, 1.6 million square feet and features two, 1000-car garages, outpatient clinical space of 400,000 square feet.

VA in Southeast Louisiana: the 30-acre main campus is part of eight community outreach clinics in the Southeast, two dental clinics and other services.

What's new: treatment for post-traumatic stress disorder, spinal cord injuries. Services for homeless veterans, chronic mental illness, substance abuse. Hospital at Home program that treats veterans in their homes, to shorten hospital stays. Tele-health programs that allow veterans to transmit personal health data from their homes.

Recent veterans: Enrollment for new programs helping recent war veterans has grown eight times since Katrina to include 4,900 veterans. Includes Mideast wars: Operations Enduring Freedom, Iraqi Freedom and New Dawn.

Area served: About 23 parishes in Southeast Louisiana.

Patients expected: 500,000 visits annually.

Staff: 1,100 new hires expected.
Source: Source: Veterans Administration May 2015. *New Orleans Times-Picayune*, March 2015

University Medical Center, New Orleans

What's in a name: The new name replaces Interim LSU Hospital. The Charity Hospital name has disappeared—except for the Spirit of Charity Trauma Center.

Location: Between Canal Street to Tulane Avenue.

Leader: Cindy Nuesslein, CEO.

What's new: The only Level 1 Trauma Center in South Louisiana, serving about 2,000 patients a year for the most serious injuries including severe traumatic brain damage and spinal cord injuries. The hospital will offer mental health services that were cut when Charity Hospital closed in 2005. A new speech therapy department. Five-story ambulatory care center. Five-story diagnostic and testing center.

Teaching hospital for: LSU New Orleans Schools of Medicine, Nursing, Dental Medicine and Allied Health. Also Tulane University School of Medicine, Xavier University, Delgado Community College, University of New Orleans, and others.

Major specialties: The hospital will treat everything from a sore throat to chronic diseases. 446 beds.

Construction budget: $1.1 billion, about $88 million short, which delayed opening.

Area served: Louisiana.

Source: University Medical Center, May 2015

Notes

Introduction
1. George Augustin. *History of Yellow Fever.* 1905. openlibrary.org., Last modified March 24, 2008. https://archive.org/stream/historyofyellow. p. 499.
2. Stephanie Stokes, "Jeff Marksmen Still Targeting Nutria," blog.nola. com. May 13, 2007. http://blog.nola.com/times-picayune/2007/05/jeff_ marksmen_still_tarketing
3. "1978: Formosan Termites Invade New Orleans," Last modified December 21, 2011, http:// www.nola.com/175 years/index. ssf/2011/12/1978_formosan_termites_invade.html
4. Bob Marshall, "Levee Leaks Reported to S&WB A Year Ago," *New*

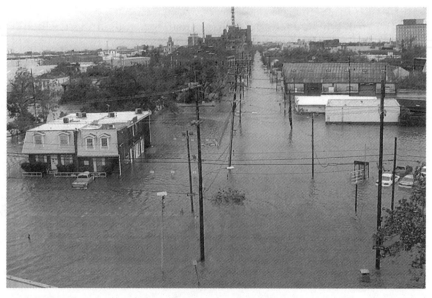

While University Hospital staff waited for help, they viewed this flood looking north along Gravier Street.

Orleans Times-Picayune, November 18, 2005, http://www.columbia.
edu/itc/journalism/cases/katrina/Press/Times-Picayune/2005-11-18

Chapter 1 Katrina Is Born

1. Select Bipartisan Committee to Investigate the Preparation for and Response to Hurricane Katrina. (2006). *A Failure of Initiative*. (2006). Washington, DC: Government Printing Office. p. 63.
2. Ibid.
3. Personal communication to author, 2015.
4. Select Bipartisan Committee, 2006, Ibid.
5. Bill Barrow, "Pendleton Memorial Methodist Hospital Settlement Leaves Disaster Planning Issues Unresolved," nola.com, accessed May 16, 2015, http://blog.nola.com/hurricane_impact/print.html?entry=/2010/01/pendleton_memorial_methodist_h_3.html
6. Select Bipartisan Committee, 2006, Ibid.
7. Select Bipartisan Committee, 2006, Ibid.
8. Robin Rudowitz, Diane Rowland, and Adele Shartzer. "Healthcare in New Orleans Before and After Hurricane Katrina." *Health Affairs*, 25, (2006).
9. Kristin Helm, Emma Eggleston, Ross Isaacs, Mohan Naddarni, Audrey Snyder, and Marcus Martin. "Into the Gap Medical Relief: Healthcare in New Orleans after Hurricane Katrina." *The Journal of Race and Policy* (2007). p. 8.
10. Ibid.
11. Personal communication, John Jones, February, 2015.
12. Ibid.
13. Personal communication, 2006.
14. Ibid.
15. CNN. *CNN Reports: Katrina—State of Emergency*. (Kansas City: Andrews & McMeel, 2005) p. 6.
16. David Bastian and Nicholas Meis. *New Orleans Hurricanes from the Start*. (Gretna: Pelican Publishing Company, 2014).
17. Warren Riley, Special Report of the Committee on Homeland Security and Governmental Affairs, US Senate. Hurricane Katrina: "A Nation Still Unprepared." (2006) Washington, DC. Government Printing Office.
18. Ibid.
19. Ibid.
20. Select Bipartisan Committee, Ibid.
21. Ibid.
22. Ibid.

23. Ibid.

Chapter 2 Axes in the Attic
1. Donald L. Canney, *In Katrina's Wake—The US Coast Guard and the Gulf Coast Hurricanes of 2005.* (Gainesville: University Press of Florida Press, 2010).
2. US Senate, Failure of Initiative, Select Bipartisan Committee to Investigate the Preparation for and Response to Hurricane Katrina, 2006 (Washington, DC: GPO).
3. Ibid., p. 26.
4. Ibid., p. 26.
5. Ibid., p. 26.
6. Ibid., p.26.
7. Canney, Ibid.
8. Ibid.
9. Ibid.
10. Ibid.
11. Warren Riley, Ibid., p. 7.
12. Ibid., p. 7.
13. Ibid., p. 7.
14. Personal communication, John Jones, 2006.
15. Douglas Brinkley. *The Great Deluge, Hurricane Katrina, New Orleans, and the Mississippi Gulf Coast.* (New York: Harper, 2007).
16. US Senate, Ibid.
17. Ibid.
18. Ibid., p. 55.
19. John McQuaid and Mark Schleifstein. *Path of Destruction—The Devastation of New Orleans and the Coming Age of Superstorms.* (New York: Little Brown, 2006) p. 212.
20. Ibid., p. 213.
21. Roger Few and Franziske (Eds.). *Flood Hazards and Health: Responding to Present and Future Risks.* (London: Cromwell, 2006).
22. US Senate, Ibid.
23. CNN, Ibid.
24. McQuaid, Ibid.
25. US Senate, Ibid.
26. Ibid.
27. Brinkley, Ibid.
28. US Senate, Ibid.
29. Personal communication, John Jones, 2006.
30. Ibid.

31. Personal communication, John Penland, 2006.
32. Ibid.
33. CNN, Ibid.
34. Ibid.
35. Ibid.

Chapter 3 Veterans Affairs Was Ready for Anything
Personal communication. 2006.

Chapter 4 Pendleton Memorial Was Closest to the Eye of the Storm
1. Personal communication. 2006.
2. Select Bipartisan Committee. Ibid.

Chapter 5 Medical Center of Louisiana in New Orleans
Personal communication, John Jones, 2006.

Chapter 6 Charity Hospital Staff Pulled Together
Personal communication, circa 2006.

Chapter 7 Tulane Medical Center Acted Decisively
1. Tulane.edu/about/history.cfm.
2. Ibid.
3. Bill Carey. *Leave No One Behind—Hurricane Katrina and the Rescue of Tulane Hospital.* (Nashville: Clearbrook Press, 2006) p. 11.
4. Ibid. p. 11.
5. Ibid. p. 19.
6. Ibid. p. 19.
7. Ibid. p. 19.
8. Personal communication. 2006.
9. Bill Carey. Ibid. p. 28.
10. Ibid.
11. Ibid.
12. Ibid., p. 112.
13. Ibid., p. 112.

Chapter 8 Ochsner Medical Center Was Well Prepared
Personal communication. 2006.

Chapter 9 Lambeth House in New Orleans Stood Tall and Strong
1. Personal communication. 2006.
2. James Cobb. *Flood of Lies—The St. Rita's Nursing Home Tragedy.*

(Gretna: Pelican Publishing Company, 2013).
3. Select Bipartisan Committee. Ibid.

Chapter 10 Emergency Operations Center
1. Select Bipartisan Committee, Ibid.
2. Ibid.
3. Ibid.
4. Ibid.
5. Ibid.
6. Ibid.
7. Personal communication. 2006.

Chapter 11 Joint Commission Recommendations for Hospital Disasters
1. Joint Commission Perspectives. *Lessons Learned from Hurricane Wilma.* (23:3, 2006).
2. Ibid.
3. Ibid.
4. Ibid.
5. Joint Commission Perspectives. Ibid.
6. NOAA, Ibid.
7. Ibid.
8. Ibid.
9. Ibid.
10. Ibid.
11. Ibid.
12. Ibid.
13. Ibid.
14. Ibid.
15. Ibid.
16. Select Bipartisan Committee. Ibid.
17. JC, Ibid.
18. Ibid.
19. Ibid.
20. Russel Honore. *Survival—How Being Prepared Can Keep You and Your Family Safe.* (New York: Simon & Shuster, 2013).
21. Ibid.
22. JC. Ibid.
23. Ibid.
24. Select Bipartisan Committee, Ibid.
25. JC. Ibid.
26. Ibid.

27. Ibid.
28. Ibid.
29. Ibid
30. Honore. Ibid.
31. Ibid.

Chapter 12 Preparing Nurses for Disaster Response

1. US Department of Labor. Bureau of Labor Statistics. January 8, 2014. http://www.bls,gov/ooh/healthcare/registered-nurses.htm
2. Christine Gebbie and Kristine Quereshi, *A Historical Challenge: Nurses and Emergencies. Online Journal of Issues in Nursing.* http://nursingworld.org/MainMenuCategories/ANAMarketplace
3. Ibid.
4. American Nurses Association. Position Paper: "Registered Nurses Rights and Responsibilities Related to Work Release During a Disaster." (2003) Washington, DC: ANA.
5. ANA. "Adapting Standards of Care under Extreme Conditions, Guidance for Professionals During Disaster, Pandemics, and Other Extreme Emergencies." (2008). Washington, DC: ANA.
6. Ibid.
7. Ibid.
8. US Department of Health & Human Services. What is ESAR-VHP? (2015) www.phe.gov/esarvhp/pages/about
9. Civilian Volunteer Medical Reserve Corps. Office of the Surgeon General. Last modified October, 2014. http://www.medicalreservecorps.gov
10. Ibid.

Chapter 13 Immediate and Long-Term Effects of Katrina

1. NBC News. "Pump Prices Jump Across US After Katrina." www.nbcnews.com/id/9146363/ns/business/t/pump-prices-jump-across-us-after-katrina
2. Personal communication. Lois. 2006.
3. Roberta Gratz. "Why Was New Orleans's Charity Hospital Allowed to Die?" *The Nation*, May 16, 2011. www.thenation.com/article/160241/why-was-new-orleans-charity-hospital-allowed to die
4. Road Home. Executive Summary: Monthly Situation & Pipeline Report #436, November 2014.
5. Personal communication.
6. Ibid.
7. Bruce Nolan. "Lindy Boggs Medical Center Purchased For Use As Nursing Home, Small Hospital." *New Orleans Times-Picayune,* May

24, 2010. www.nola.com/news/index.ssf/2010/o5/catholic_non-proft_buys_lindy.html

8. Bruce Nolan. "New Hospitals Revive Faith-Based Traditions." *New Orleans Times-Picayune,* April 9, 2012.

9. Ibid.

10. US Department of Veterans Affairs. PTSD: National Center for PTSD. www.ptsd.va.gov/professional/index.asp

11. American Psychological Association. *Diagnostic and Statistical Manual IV.* p. 467

12. Ibid.

13. Ibid.

14. Ibid.

15. Veterans Affairs. Ibid.

16. Wendy Park. "Nurse's Posttraumatic Stress, Level of Exposure, and Coping Five Years After Hurricane Katrina." (PhD dissertation, Georgia State University, October, 2011).

17. Ibid.

18. H. Osofsky and Osofsky, Arey, Kronenberg, Hansel, and Many (2011). "Hurricane Katrina's First Responders: the Struggle to Protect and Serve in the Aftermath of Disaster." www.ncbi.min.nih.gov

19. K. McLaughlin, P. Berglund, M. Gruber, R. Kessler, N. Samson, and A. Zaskavsky, (2011). "Recovery from PTSD Following Hurricane Katrina. Depression and Anxiety." 28(6): 439-446.

20. Personal communication.

21. Southeast Flood Protection Authority. slfpa.org/resources/facts2006. Last updated 2015.

22. NOAA, Ibid.

23. American Society of Civil Engineers. "The New Orleans Hurricane Protection System: What Went Wrong and Why." cms.asce.org 2006.

24. American Society, Ibid.

25. Ibid.

26. US Court of Appeals. US Corps of Engineers.

Bibliography

"1978: Formosan Termites Invade New Orleans," Last modified December 21, 2011, http://www.nola.com/175 years/index.ssf/2011/12/1978_formosan_termites_invade.html

American Psychological Association. *Diagnostic and Statistical Manual IV*. p. 467.

American Society of Civil Engineers. "The New Orleans Hurricane Protection System: What Went Wrong and Why." 2006.

American Nurses Association. Position Paper: "Registered Nurses Rights and Responsibilities Related to Work Release During a Disaster." (2003) Washington, DC: ANA.

American Nurses Association. "Adapting Standards of Care Under Extreme Conditions, Guidance for Professionals During Disaster, Pandemics, and Other Extreme Emergencies." (2008). Washington, DC: ANA.

Augustin, G., (1906). *History of Yellow Fever*. openlibrary.org. Last modified March 24, 2008. https://archive.org/stream/historyofyellowfever

Bastian, D. F., Meis, D. J. *New Orleans Hurricanes from the Start*. (Gretna: Pelican Publishing Company, 2014).

Brinkley, D. *The Great Deluge—Hurricane Katrina, New Orleans, and the Mississippi Gulf Coast*. (New York: Harper, 2007).

Broder, John "Scientists See More Deadly Weather, But Dispute The Cause." *New York Times*. June 16, 2011, http://www.nytimes.com/2011/06/16/science /earth/16climate.html

Civilian Volunteer Medical Reserve Corps. Office of the Surgeon General. Last modified October, 2014. http://www.medicalreservecorps.gov

CNN. *Katrina—State of Emergency*. (Kansas City: Andrews & McMeel, 2005).

Center for Disease Control and Prevention. "Public Health Response to Hurricanes Katrina and Rita—Louisiana, 2005." March 10, 2006. MMWR 55 (9): 29-30.

Center for Disease Control and Prevention. "Assessment of Health-Related Needs After Hurricanes Katrina and Rita—Orleans and Jefferson Parishes, New Orleans Area, Louisiana October, 17-22, 2005" (2006). MMWR 55 (9): 38-41.

Gebbie, C. and Qureshi, K. *"A Historical Challenge: Nurses and Emergencies." Online Journal of Nursing.* (2006).

Gratz, Roberta. "Why Was New Orleans's Charity Hospital Allowed to Die?" *The Nation.* May 16, 2011. www.thenation.com/article/160241/why-was-new-orleans-charity-hospital-allowed-to die.

Greater New Orleans Expressway Commission, Lake Ponchartrain Causeway Bridge. Accessed January 22, 2014. http://www.thecauseway.us/causeway/commission.php .

Helm, K., Eggleston, E., Isaacs, R., Nadkarni, M., Snyder, A., Martin, M. "Into the Gap Medical Relief: Healthcare in New Orleans After Hurricane Katrina." *The Journal of Race and Policy* 2007. 3:132-140.

Horne, Jed. *Hurricane Katrina and the Near Death of a Great American City.* (New York. Random House. 2006).

Joint Commission. *Joint Commission Perspectives. Lessons Learned from Hurricane Wilma.* March, 2006. 26-3, p. 5-8.

Louisiana Health Report Card. (2005). Submitted to the Governor and the Louisiana Legislature March, 2006. www.dhh.louisiana.gov/reports.asp

Louisiana Recovery Authority. Quarterly Report: February-May 2006. Retrieved from http//www.Ira.louisiana.gov/assets/quarterlyreport/LRAQarterlyReport060606pdf.pdf

Marshall, Bob. "Levee Leaks Reported to S&WB A Year Ago," *New Orleans Times-Picayune,* November 18, 2005, accessed Jan 27, 2015. http://www.columbia.edu/itc/journalism/cases/katrina/Press/Times-Picayune/2005-\11-18

Marshall, B., Swenson, D. *Flash Flood, Hurricane Katrina's Inundation of New Orleans, August 29, 2005* [Electronic version]. Retrieved November 1, 2011, from National Weather Service. (2005, August). Katrina Graphics Archive. Retrieved November 1, 2011 from http://www.nhc.noaa.gov/archive/2005/katrina_graphics.shtml

McQuaid, J. and Schleifstein, Mark. *Path to Destruction—The Devastation of New Orleans and the Coming Age of Superstorms.* (New York: Little, Brown & Co., 2006).

NOAA, US Department of Commerce, National Oceanic and Atmospheric Administration. *Extreme Weather 2011.* Last modified January 19, 2012.

Nolan, Bruce "Lindy Boggs Medical Center Purchased For Use As Nursing

Home, Small Hospital. *" New Orleans Times-Picayune,* May 24, 2010.

Nolan, B. "New Hospitals Revive Faith-Based Traditions." *New Orleans Times-Picayune.* April 9, 2012.

Office of the US Surgeon General. Civilian Volunteer Medical Reserve Corps. Accessed October 14, 2014. http://www.medicalreservecorps.gov

Riley, Warren. Senate Committee on Homeland Security and Governmental Affairs. *Testimony of the Superintendent of the New Orleans Police Department.* (2006).

Road Home. Executive Summary: Monthly Situation & Pipeline Report #436, November 2014.

Robertson, Campbell and Schwartz, John. "Decade After Katrina, Pointing Finger More Firmly at Army Corps." *New York Times,* May 24, 2015. http://www.nytimes.com/2015/05/24decade-after-katrina-pointing-finger-more-firmly-at-army-corps

Rudowitz, R., Rowland, D., Shartzer, A. "Healthcare in New Orleans Before And After Hurricane Katrina." *Health Affairs. 2006* 25: 393-406.

Salvaggio, J. *New Orleans' Charity Hospital: A Story of Physicians, Politics, and Poverty.* (Baton Rouge: LSU Press, 1992).

Select Bipartisan Committee to Investigate the Preparation for and Response to Hurricane Katrina. "A Failure of Initiative." (2006). Washington, DC: Government Printing Office.

Special Report of the Committee on Homeland Security and Governmental Affairs, US Senate. (2006). "Hurricane Katrina: A Nation Still Unprepared." Washington, DC: Government Printing Office.

Stokes, Stephanie. "Jeff Marksmen Still Targeting Nutria," blog.nola.com. May13, 2007. Accessed January 27, 2015. http://blog.nola.com/times-picayune/2007/05/jeff_marksmen_still_targeting

US Department of Labor. Bureau of Labor Statistics. Wednesday January 8, 2014. http://www.bls,gov/ooh/healthcare/registered-nurses.htm

US Department of Veterans Affairs. PTSD: National Center for PTSD. www.ptsd.va.gov/professional/index.asp

Wilds, John *Oschner's—An Informal History of the South's Largest Private Medical Center.* (Baton Rouge: LSU Press, 1985).

Index